WEIGHT WATCHERS

By Michael Collins

Slow Cooker Smart Points Cookbook, Discover Rapid & Healthy Weight Loss, "Set & Forget" To Lose Fat Fast The Natural Way

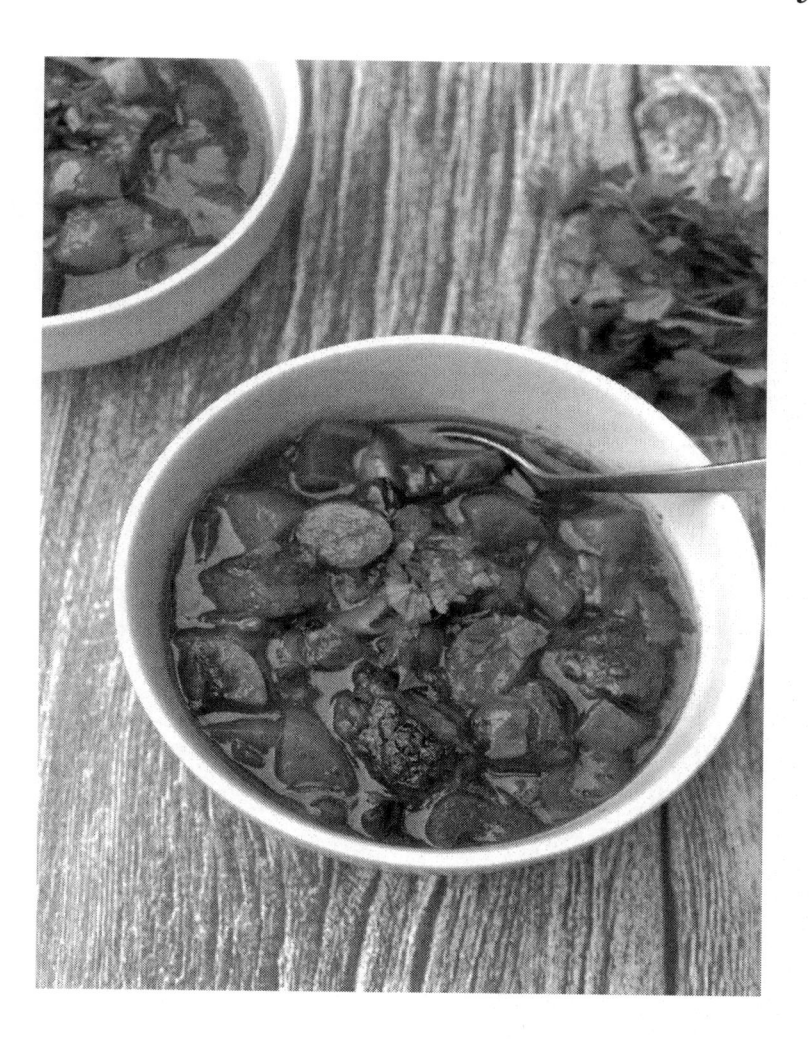

@ Copyright 2017 by Michael Collins All rights reserved.
In no way is it legal to reproduce, duplicate, or transmit any part of this document in either electronic means or in printed format. Recording of this publication is strictly prohibited and any storage of this document is not allowed unless with written permission from the publisher. All rights reserved.

The information provided herein is stated to be truthful and consistent, in that any liability, in terms of inattention or otherwise, by any usage or abuse of any policies, processes, or directions contained within is the solitary and utter responsibility of the recipient reader. Under no circumstances will any legal responsibility or blame be held against the publisher for any reparation, damages, or monetary loss due to the information herein, either directly or indirectly.

Respective authors own all copyrights not held by the publisher.
The information herein is offered for informational purposes solely, and is universal as so. The

presentation of the information is without contract or any type of guarantee assurance.

The trademarks that are used are without any consent, and the publication of the trademark is without permission or backing by the trademark owner. All trademarks and brands within this book are for clarifying purposes only and are the owned by the owners themselves, not affiliated with this document.

Table of Contents

Introduction 8
Chapter1: What Are "Smart Points" 9
The Do's And Don't: 12
Chapter 2: What Is Slow Cooker 14
    Benefits Of Using A slow Cooker 15
Chapter 3: Slow Cooker Smart points Soup & Stew Recipes 17
    Delicious Chicken Noodle Soup 18
    Creamy Onion Parmesan Tomato Soup 20
    Creamy Garlic Potato Cauliflower 22
    Chili Onion Double-Bean Beef Soup 23
    Delicious Spicy Turkey Stew 24
    Spicy Garlic Corn Bean Pork 25
    Tasty Rosemary Thyme Beef Stew 27
    Delicious Ham Milk Rice Soup 29
    Coconut Carrot Ginger Soup 30
    Spicy Tomato Ginger Peanut Soup 32
    French Onion Soup 34
    Cumin Garlic Spiced Beans 35
    Delicious Squash Soup 36
    Kale and Corn Soup 37
    Delicious Special Veggie Stew 38
    Healthy Mushroom Spinach Gnocchi Soup 39
Chapter 4: Slow Cooker Smart Points Chicken & Turkey Recipes
.... 40
    Lime Garlic Chicken 40
    Mushroom Cinnamon Chicken 42
    Brussels Sprouts Ginger Mustard Chicken 44

Tomato Mushroom Chicken 46

Feta Olive Artichoke Chicken 47

Yummy Cumin Jalapeno Chicken 48

Delicious Garlic Celery Buffalo Chicken 49

Lemon Garlic Herbs Chicken 50

Italian Style Balsamic Chicken 51

Delicious Mexican Style Casserole 52

Tasty Savory Apple Chicken 54

Simple Chili Chicken 55

Chicken Meatloaf 56

Delicious Barbecue Turkey 58

Pinto Beans Bay Leaf Turkey 59

Cheesy Eggplant Eggplant Chicken 60

Yummy Curry Chicken 61

Chapter 5: Slow Cooker Smart points Beef &Pork Recipes 62

Yummy Pulled Pork 63

Garlic Worcestershire Sauce Braised Beef 64

Beef Taco Filling 65

Thyme Ginger Apricots Pork Chops 66

Yummy Chili Taco Filling 67

Tasty Mushroom Pork Meatloaf 69

Mustard Chili Garlic Beef Ribs 71

Cashew Coconut Tenderloin 72

Jalapeno Ginger Beef in Sauce 73

Yummy Shredded Beef 74

Delight Roast Beef 76

Onion Chili Beef Roast Tacos 77

Delicious Stuffed Flank Roll 78

Champagne Slow Cooker Sauerbraten ... 80
Delicious Coconut Curry Beef ... 82
Tasty Beef Stew ... 83
Spicy Oregano Pulled Pork ... 84
Spicy Tumeric Honey Pork Chops ... 85
Apple Pork Tenderloin ... 86
Ginger Spices Hoisin Pork ... 87
Shallots Spinach Pork Tenderloin ... 88
Sesame Ginger Onion Pork ... 90
Garlic Sweet and Sour Pork ... 91

Chapter 6: Slow Cooker Smart Points Vegetarian Recipes ... 92
Yummy Black Bean Enchiladas with Spinach ... 93
Delicious Vegetable Fusion ... 95
Tasty Polenta and Beans ... 96
Garlic Vegan Chili ... 97
Squash Soup ... 98
Shallots Pumpkin Braised Stew ... 99
Onion Split Pea Soup ... 100
Slow Cooker Stuffed Peppers ... 101
Roasted Potatoes ... 103
Three Bean Chili ... 104
Lentil and Pumpkin Stew ... 105
Healthy Vegan Stew ... 106
Special Slow Cooker Risotto ... 107
Cinnamon Squash and Apples Mix ... 109
Sweet Potato Soup ... 110
Mushroom Vegan Cassoulet ... 111
Potato Chowder ... 112

Soy Sauce Marinated Mushrooms 113
Minestrone Soup 114
Yummy Sweet Vegetable Lasagna 115
Thyme French Onion Soup 117
Delicious Mexican Fried Beans 118
Conclusion: 119

Introduction

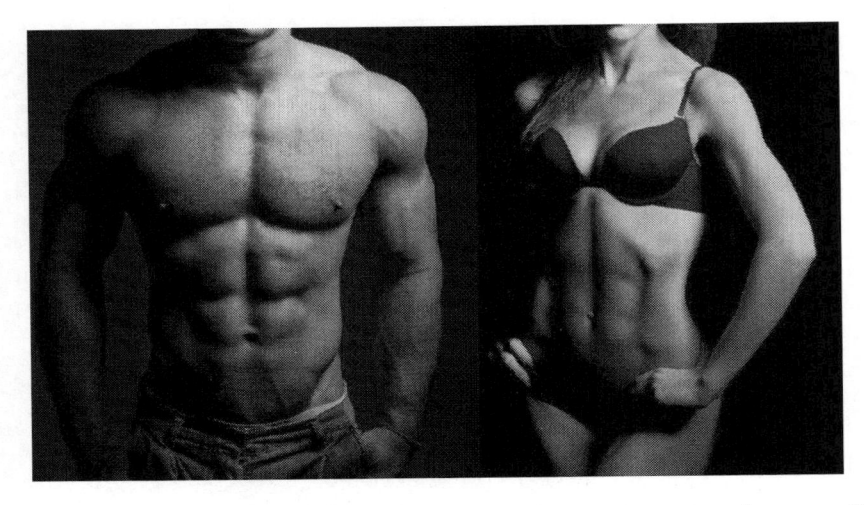

Congratulation and thank you for your purchase of my book, *"Weight Watchers: Slow Cooker Smart Points Cookbook, Discover Rapid & Healthy Weight Loss, "Set & Forget" To Lose Fat Fast The Natural Way.*

Weight Watchers diet is tracked using a **point-based system**, and this book contains proven steps and strategies on how to lose weight effectively, and stay healthy and happy

Chapter 1: What Are "Smart Points"

The SmartPoints system is the latest revision of the Weight Watchers system.

The designers of the SmartPoints system use the economy of points to make weight loss simple, while still including much of the complex nutritional information of these foods into a simple singular number.

Smart Points is a simple and easy system to follow. It is an improvement from older systems and more effective accordingly as well.

For instance, foods that have a high content of saturated fat or sugar have a high SmartPoints value.

Food that has a high content of lean protein has lower SmartPoints value.

The lower valued SmartPoints food is actually healthier. So you see how you get healthier by the day as you make better choices in what you eat.

Once you join the program, you get a personalized budget of SmartPoints. It includes a daily and weekly budget along with guides on how to keep track of when you eat too much, like at restaurants. You will be provided with some easy tools that will help you with all this.

The SmartPoints option will allow you to eat anything you like as long as you follow the points budget.

Anything else is off your diet.

You will just get a chance to eat a few of those treats that aren't on the diet like an allowance each week. So you can go for the Smart Points system to eat whatever you like or go for a more drastic change in diet with the No Count system. Either way, Weight Watchers will help you reach the weight loss goal you have set.

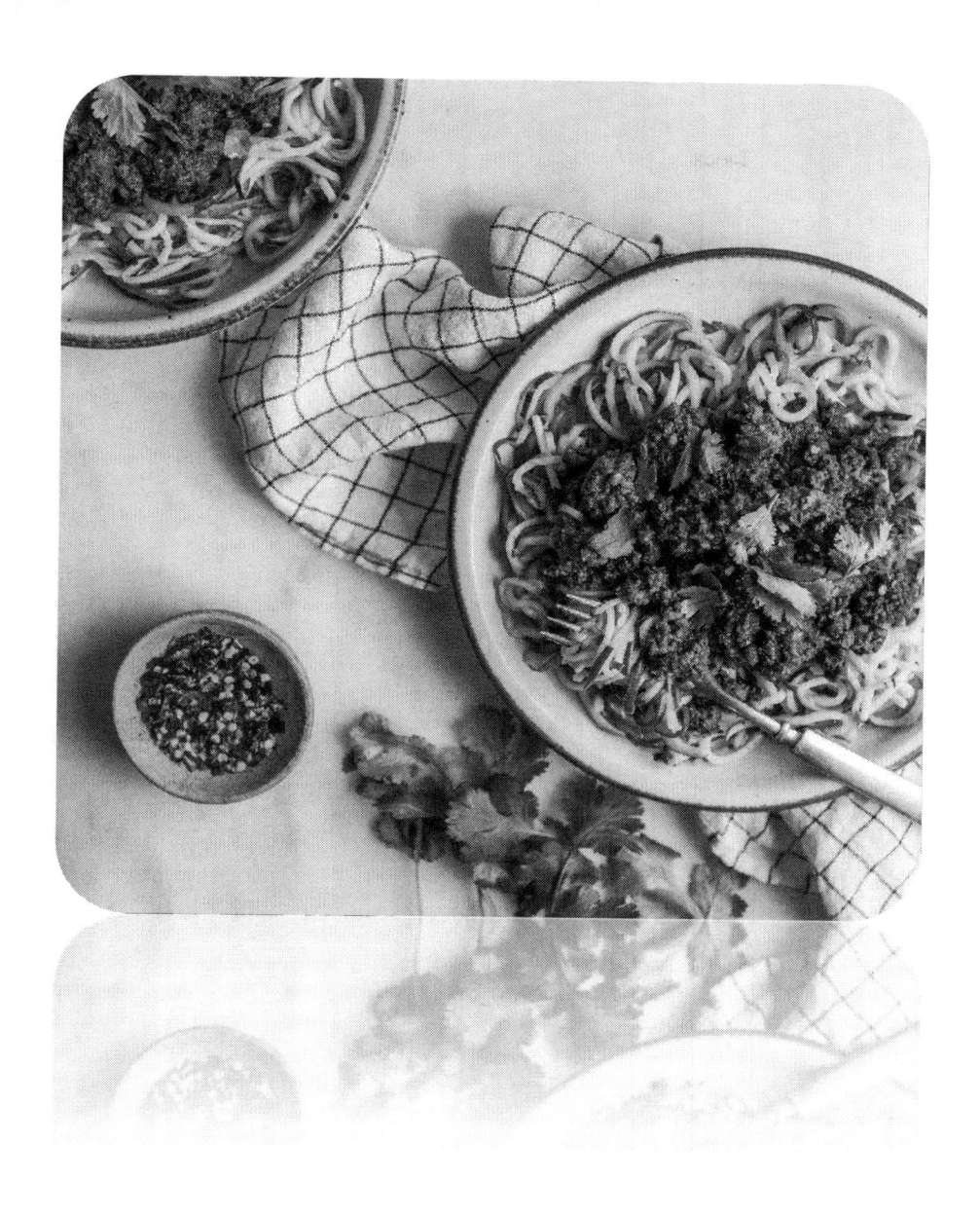

The Do's And Don't:

Things to avoid when you follow the points system:

- Do not try to guess the point values of what you eat. You also cannot use the old point's calculator if you want the results for the new program. Do not think that just noting the calorie value on labels of foods will work the same as using the point's calculator.

The Points Plus values are calculated differently and are meant to help you stay full without eating excessively. It notes down how much energy will be available in your body once you eat the food and this will depend on exactly what you eat.

- Do not try to combine the different programs, as this won't be effective. Follow your specific program and follow all steps in it rigorously.

Use the point's calculator to keep track of this and not go off base.

- Do not try to trick the system. If you eat a little less on one day and do not reach your target point for the day, it does not mean you can eat more the next day. Those points do not get added to the next day target.

It is important that you track the portion size properly for the Points Plus value to show correctly. This will make a difference in your daily target. Being lazy will just push you off track from your progress.

- Please note: Just because something is healthy does not mean you can over eat it. Too much of nothing is good for your body. Fruits, for instance, are something that you should definitely eat every day. Eat so that it keeps you full and you do not crave anything unhealthy.

Portion size matters for fruits as well. Some fruits, in particular, have a high calorific value. So keep this in mind and eat mindfully.

Chapter 2: What Is Slow Cooker

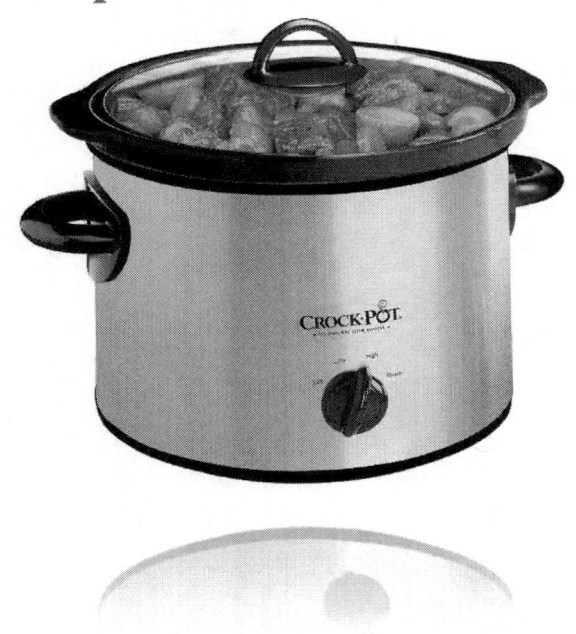

Slow cooking is a method of creating a meal using a countertop device called a 'slow-cooker'; a machine that uses electricity to heat up the ceramic bowl inside. It is topped with a glass lid and uses a low-heat setting to prepare food over a long period of time.

The slow cooker is specially designed to handle so-called 'one-pot' meals, which don't need as much meal prep compared to conventional cooking methods. This way, ingredients can be chopped into larger chunks, add a bit of your favorite seasoning, any liquids your meal might need, and that is all

Benefits Of Using A slow Cooker

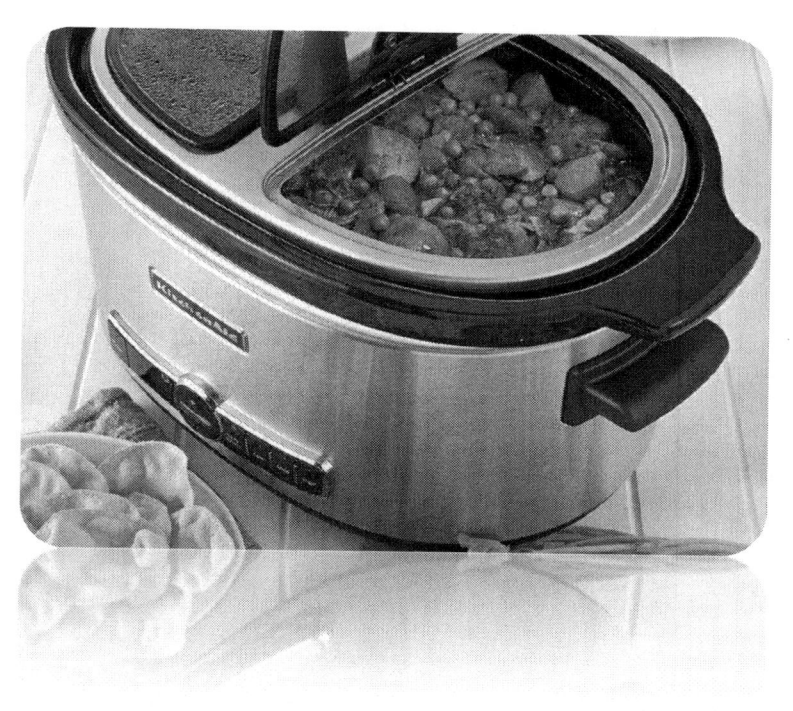

- Affordable
- Super Convenient
- Energy Efficiency
- Ideal for cook almost all types of food
- Very simple to use
- Clean & Pleasant etc

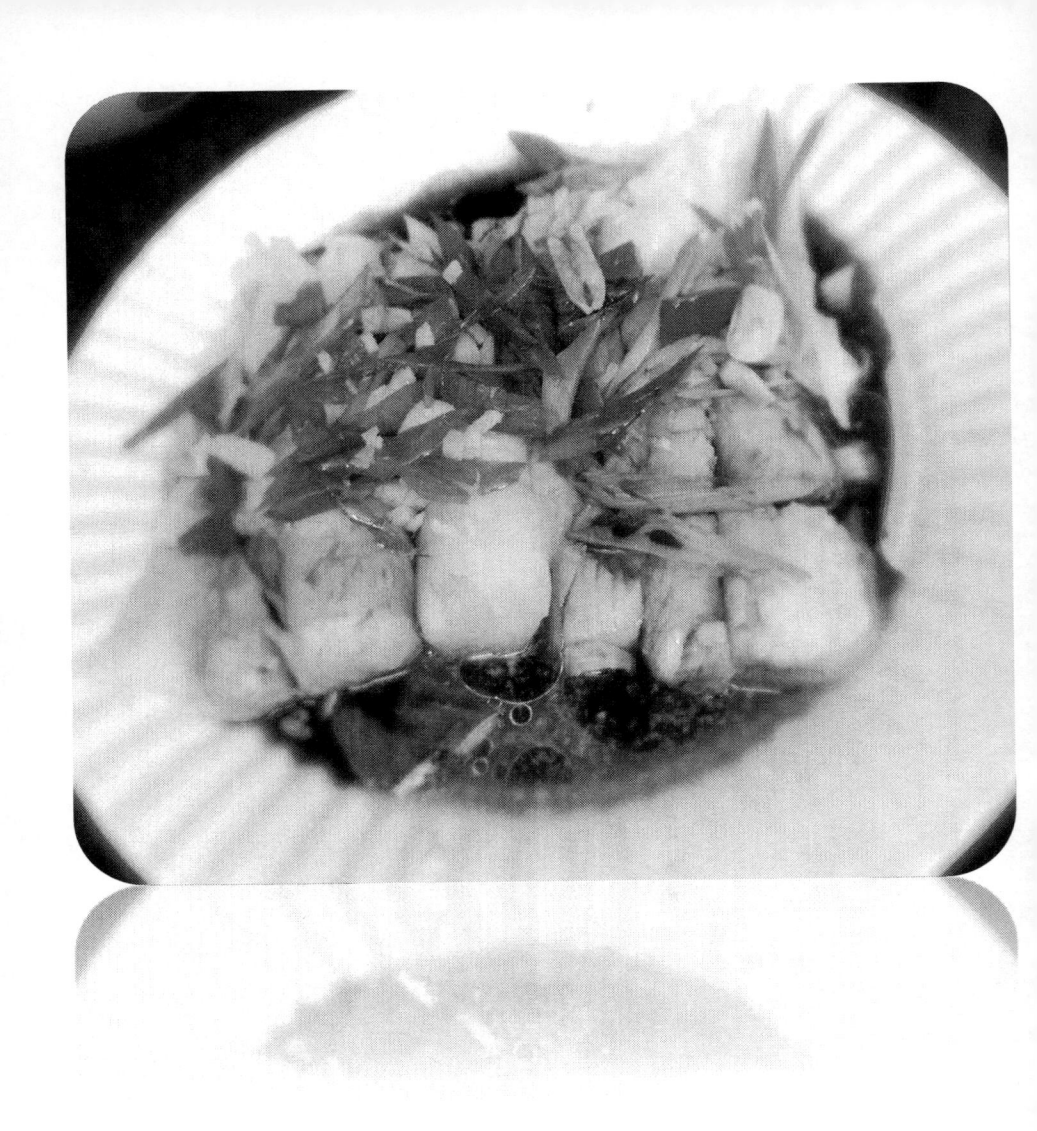

Chapter 3: Slow Cooker Smart points Soup & Stew Recipes

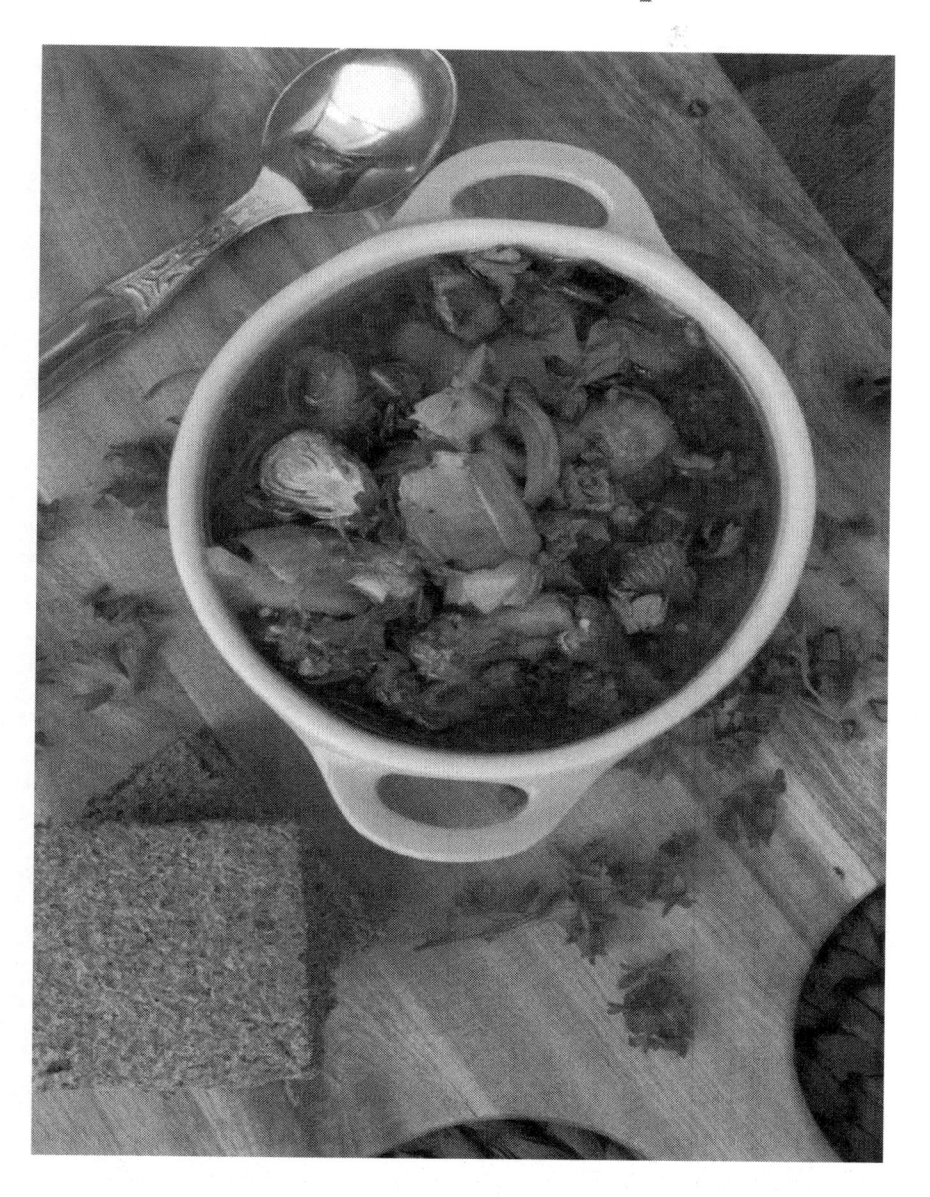

Delicious Chicken Noodle Soup

Serves: 8

Smart Points: 6

Ingredients:

- 2 pounds bone in chicken pieces, skin removed
- 1 tablespoon olive oil
- 2 cups carrots, chopped
- 2 cups celery, chopped
- 1 cup yellow onion, chopped
- 2 cloves garlic, crushed and minced
- 1 tablespoon tomato pasted
- ½ teaspoon salt
- 1 teaspoon black pepper
- 8 cups chicken broth
- 2 bay leaves
- 1 sprig fresh rosemary
- 1 tablespoon fresh thyme, chopped
- ½ pound egg noodles, cooked
- ¼ cup fresh parsley, chopped

Directions:

1. Heat the olive oil in a skillet over medium heat.
2. Once the pan is hot, add the chicken pieces and cook until browned on all sides. This should take approximately 5-7 minutes.
3. Remove the chicken from the skillet and place it directly into the slow cooker.

4. Add the carrots, celery and onion to the remaining oil in the skillet. Sauté the vegetables over medium heat until tender, approximately 5 minutes.

5. Add in the garlic, tomato paste, salt and black pepper. Cook, stirring frequently for 3-5 minutes.

6. Add one cup of the chicken stock to the skillet and scrape any browned bits from the pan. Transfer the vegetable and sauce mixture to the slow cooker with the chicken.

7. Next, add the remaining chicken broth, bay leaves, rosemary and thyme to the slow cooker.

8. Cover and cook on low for 6 hours.

9. Remove the cover and shred the chicken, making sure to remove all of the bones from the soup. Add in the cooked egg noodles and fresh parsley.

10. Stir and cook an additional 30 minutes before serving.

Nutrition Value: Calories 276, Fat 4 g, Carbs 28 g, Protein 30 g

Creamy Onion Parmesan Tomato Soup

Smart Points: 6

Ingredients:

- 1 tablespoon olive oil
- 2 14-ounce cans stewed tomatoes
- 4 roma tomatoes, quartered
- 1 cup sweet yellow onion, diced
- 1 tablespoon brown sugar
- 1 tablespoon tomato paste
- 2 cloves garlic, crushed and minced
- 1/2 teaspoon salt
- 1 teaspoon coarse ground black pepper
- 2 tablespoons flour
- 1/4 cup fresh basil, chopped
- 3 cups vegetable broth
- 1 cup plain, unsweetened almond milk
- ¼ cup fresh grated parmesan cheese

Directions:

1. Heat the olive oil in a skillet over medium heat.
2. Add in the stewed tomatoes, roma tomatoes, and sweet yellow onion. Sauté the mixture for 4-6 minutes, or until the roma tomatoes begin to blister and break apart.
3. Next, add in the brown sugar, tomato paste, garlic, salt and coarse ground black pepper. Cook, stirring frequently for 3 minutes.

4. Add in the flour and cook for 1 minute while stirring or whisking to break apart any lumps.

5. Remove the skillet from the heat and transfer the mixture to a slow cooker.

6. Add in the fresh basil and vegetable broth.

7. Cover and cook on low for 7 hours.

8. Remove the cover and transfer one half of the soup mixture to a blender and puree until smooth. Transfer the contents back into the slow cooker. If you would like a soup with a creamier texture, puree all of the contents of the slow cooker.

9. Next, add in the almond milk and parmesan cheese.

10. Cover and cook an additional 45 minutes before serving.

Nutrition Value: Calories 143, Fat 5 g, Carbs 25 g, Protein 4 g

Creamy Garlic Potato Cauliflower

Smart Points: 2

Servings: 8

Ingredients:
- Salt
- Ground pepper
- Grated parmesan cheese
- 4 cups of water
- 4 garlic cloves
- 3 cups of vegetable broth
- 1 tablespoon of olive oil
- 2 medium potatoes, peeled and cubed
- 2 cauliflower heads

Directions:
1. Place all the ingredients in the slow cooker. Cook on low for about five hours.
2. Let the soup cool and then place into the blender. Process for about 2 minutes.
3. Serve and enjoy.

Nutrition Value: Calories 97, Fat 5 g, Carbs 15 g, Protein 5.1 g

Chili Onion Double-Bean Beef Soup

Smart Points: 5

Servings: 8

Ingredients:

- 1 tablespoon of chili powder
- 1 tablespoon of cumin
- 1 pack of taco seasoning
- 1 cup of frozen corn
- 1 ½ cups of chopped onion
- 1 can of tomato sauce
- 1 can of black beans
- 1 can of kidney beans
- 1 can of diced tomatoes
- 1 pound of extra lean ground beef

Directions:

1. Heat some olive oil in a nonstick pan. Cook beef for about 10 minutes. Remove from heat.
2. Place the cooked meat in the slow cooker. Add the tomato sauce, onions, taco seasoning, corn, chili, cumin, and beans.
3. Cover and cook on high for five hours. Serve and enjoy.

Nutrition Value: Calories 230, Fat: 2g, Carbs 36 g, Protein 23 g

Delicious Spicy Turkey Stew

Serves: 6

SmartPoints: 6

Ingredients:

- 1 ½ pounds turkey breast, cut into quarters
- 1 teaspoon salt
- 1 teaspoon black pepper
- 1 tablespoon chili powder
- 1 cup red onion, diced
- 2 tablespoons jalapeno pepper, diced
- 4 cloves garlic, crushed and minced
- 1 tablespoon tomato paste
- 4 cups chicken broth
- 1 tablespoon honey
- 2 cups tomatoes, chopped
- 2 cups yellow hominy
- 1 cup black beans, cooked
- ¼ cup chipotle pepper in adobo sauce, chopped
- ¼ cup fresh cilantro, chopped

Directions:

1. Season the turkey breast with salt, black pepper, and chili powder. Place the turkey breasts in the bottom of a slow cooker.
2. Next, add in the red onion, jalapeno pepper, and garlic.
3. Whisk together the tomato paste, chicken broth, and honey in a glass bowl. Pour the liquid into the slow cooker.
4. To the slow cooker, add in the tomatoes, yellow hominy, black beans, and chipotle pepper with the adobo sauce.
5. Cover and cook on low for 8 hours.

6. Remove the cover and shred the turkey.
7. Garnish the stew with fresh cilantro before serving.

Nutrition Value: Calories 272, Fat 4 g, Carbs 25 g, Protein 33 g

Spicy Garlic Corn Bean Pork

Serves: 6

Smart Points: 8

Ingredients:

- 1 ½ pounds tomatillos
- 1 cup yellow onion, diced
- 5 cloves garlic, crushed and minced
- 2 tablespoons olive oil
- 1 teaspoon cumin
- ¼ teaspoon cinnamon
- ¼ teaspoon cayenne powder
- 2 cups fresh corn kernels
- 3 cups chicken broth
- 1 cup poblano pepper, chopped
- 1 pound pork tenderloin, cubed
- ½ teaspoon salt
- 1 teaspoon black pepper
- 1 teaspoon Mexican oregano
- 1 cup canned white beans, rinsed
- Fresh cilantro for garnish, optional
- Cooked rice for serving, optional

Directions:

1. Begin by preheating the broiler of your oven and line a baking sheet with aluminum foil.
2. Next, remove the husks from the tomatillos, cut them in half and place them in a bowl.
3. Add the onions and garlic to the tomatillos and stir.
4. Drizzle the olive oil over the tomatillos and season the mixture with the cumin, cinnamon, and cayenne pepper. Toss to coat.
5. Spread the tomatillos mixture out onto the foil lined baking sheet. Place the baking sheet under the broiler for 7-10 minutes, stirring once halfway through.
6. Remove baking sheet from the broiler and let the tomatillos cool slightly.
7. Once cooled, transfer the roasted vegetables to a blender or food processor and blend until smooth.
8. Transfer the mixture to a slow cooker and add in the corn kernels, poblano peppers, and chicken broth.
9. Season the pork with the salt, black pepper, and Mexican oregano.
10. Add the pork, along with the white beans to the slow cooker.
11. Cover and cook on low for 6 hours.
12. Serve garnished with fresh cilantro, over cooked rice, if desired.

Nutrition Value: Calories 292, Fat 13 g, Carbs 21 g, Protein 26 g

Tasty Rosemary Thyme Beef Stew

SmartPoints: 6

Servings: 8

Ingredients:

- 1 sprig of thyme
- 1 sprig of rosemary
- 2 cups of beef broth
- 2 tablespoons of cornstarch
- ¼ teaspoon of ground allspice
- 1 teaspoon of smoked paprika
- ½ teaspoon of pepper
- 1 teaspoon of brown sugar
- 1 ½ teaspoons of salt
- 2 bay leaves
- 1 garlic clove, minced
- 2 whole garlic cloves
- 2 cups of water
- 1 tablespoon of olive oil
- 2 tablespoons of Worcestershire sauce
- 1 diced onion
- 3 celery ribs, chopped
- 1 pound of chopped red potatoes
- ½ pound chopped parsnips
- ½ pound chopped carrots
- 1 ½ pounds of lean stewing beef (cut into chunks)

Directions:

1. Heat the olive oil in a large soup pot over medium heat.
2. Add the beef and cook for five minutes each side.

3.   Add the thyme, rosemary, smoked paprika, garlic, onion, water, Worcestershire sauce, pepper, salt, sugar, and allspice.

4.   Cover and simmer for about 90 minutes

5.   Add carrots, potatoes, celery, parsnips, and beef broth. Cook for about an hour.

Nutrition Value: Calories 233, Fat 6 g, Carbs 24 g, Protein 22g

Delicious Ham Milk Rice Soup

Nutrition Value: Calories 205, Fat 8 g, Carbs 20 g, Protein 13g

SmartPoints: 5

Servings: 8

Ingredients:

- ½ cup of evaporated milk
- ¼ teaspoon of ground black pepper
- 1 can of cream of celery soup
- 2 cups of chicken broth
- 3 cups of water
- 1 pack of mixed vegetable
- ¾ cup of uncooked wild rice
- ½ cup of chopped onion
- 2 cups of diced cooked ham

Directions:

1. Combine all the ingredients in the slow cooker, except the milk.
2. Cook on low for seven hours.
3. Stir in the milk and cook for another ten minutes.

Nutrition Value: Calories 205, Fat 8 g, Carbs 20 g, Protein 13g

Coconut Carrot Ginger Soup

Serves: 6

SmartPoints: 5

Ingredients:

- 6 cups carrots, chopped
- 1 cup onion, diced
- 2 cloves garlic, crushed and minced
- 2 teaspoons olive oil
- 2 tablespoons fresh grated ginger
- ¼ teaspoon cayenne pepper powder
- ½ teaspoon salt
- 1 teaspoon black pepper
- 1 tablespoon honey
- 4 cups vegetable broth
- ¼ cup flour
- ¼ cup fresh orange juice
- 1 cup coconut milk

Directions:

1. Combine the carrots, onion, and garlic in a slow cooker.
2. Drizzle the vegetables with the olive oil and then add the fresh grated ginger cayenne pepper powder, salt, and black pepper. Mix well.
3. Whisk together the vegetable broth and the honey in a separate bowl. Add the broth into the slow cooker.
4. Cover and cook on low for 6 hours.
5. Transfer the soup to a blender, working in batches if necessary, and puree until smooth. Return the soup back to the slow cooker.
6. Whisk together the flour, orange juice, and coconut milk in separate bowl.

7. Add the liquid to the slow cooker with the soup and mix well.

8. Replace the cover on the slow cooker; increase the heat to high and cook an additional 45 minutes before serving.

Nutrition Value: Calories 124, Fat 2 g, Carbs 24g, Protein 2g

Spicy Tomato Ginger Peanut Soup

Serves: 10

SmartPoints: 7

Ingredients:

- 1 tablespoon olive oil
- 1 cup yellow onion, diced
- 1 cup red bell pepper, diced
- 1 cup sweet potato, diced
- 4 cloves garlic, crushed and minced
- 1 14-ounce can roasted tomatoes, with liquid
- 1 cup uncooked couscous
- 6 cups vegetable broth
- 1 cup coconut milk
- 1 tablespoon fresh grated ginger
- 1 tablespoon low sodium soy sauce
- 1 tablespoon lime juice
- 1 teaspoon chili powder
- 1 teaspoon curry powder
- 1 teaspoon white pepper
- ½ teaspoon salt
- ¾ cup sugar free natural peanut butter
- ¼ cup chopped peanut for garnish

Directions:

1. Heat the olive oil in a skillet over medium heat.
2. Add the yellow onion, red bell pepper, and sweet potatoes to the skillet. Cook, stirring frequently, for 5 minutes.
3. Transfer the contents of the skillet into the slow cooker.

4. Next, add in the garlic, roasted tomatoes, couscous, vegetable broth, coconut milk, ginger, low sodium soy sauce, lime juice, chili powder, curry powder, white pepper, and salt. Mix well.

5. Cover and cook on low for 7 hours.

6. Remove the cover and stir in the peanut butter. Return the cover and cook and additional 30 minutes.

7. Serve garnished with chopped peanuts.

Nutrition Value: Calories 240, Fat 12 g, Carbs 25g, Protein 8g

French Onion Soup

SmartPoints: 3

Servings: 8

Ingredients:

- 2 tablespoons of thyme
- 2 cups of vegetable broth
- 3 tablespoons of all-purpose flour
- ½ teaspoon of salt
- ½ teaspoon of pepper
- 2 tablespoons of brown sugar
- 3 garlic cloves, minced
- 1 tablespoon of balsamic vinegar
- 1 tablespoon of Worcestershire sauce
- 2 tablespoons of butter
- 4 sweet onions, sliced

Directions:

1. Place the butter, onion, vinegar, Worcestershire sauce, garlic, pepper, brown sugar, and salt in the slow cooker. Cook on high for one hour.
2. Add the flour and cook for another five minutes.
3. Add the thyme and the broth, and cook on low for six hours.
4. Serve with cheese and bread.

Nutrition Value: Calories 111, Fat 3 g, Carbs 20g, Protein 2g

Cumin Garlic Spiced Beans

SmartPoints: 4

Servings: 8

Ingredients:
- 6 cups of water
- 2 bay leaves
- 1 teaspoon of salt
- ½ tablespoon of cumin
- 2 poblano peppers, diced
- 4 garlic cloves, diced
- 1 onion, diced
- 1 pound of pinto beans, rinsed

Directions:
1. Add all the ingredients in the crackpot.
2. Cook on low for about seven hours.

Nutrition Value: Calories 129, Fat 1 g, Carbs 37g, Protein 14g

Delicious Squash Soup

SmartPoints: 6

Servings: 6

Ingredients:
- 4 cups of vegetable broth
- 1 butternut squash, chopped
- 3 garlic cloves, minced
- 3 carrots, chopped
- 1 onion, chopped

Directions:
1. Add all the ingredients in the slow cooker.
2. Cook on low for seven hours.
3. Place in a blender and process for a few minutes.
4. Serve and enjoy.

Nutrition Value: Calories 62, Fat 0 g, Carbs 15g, Protein 2g

Kale and Corn Soup

SmartPoints: 4

Servings: 6

Ingredients:
- Pepper
- Salt
- 2 teaspoons of chili powder
- 2 teaspoons of oregano
- 2 teaspoons of cumin
- 1 bay leaf
- 4 garlic cloves, minced
- 4 cups of chopped kale
- 1 onion, minced
- 1 can of regular corn
- 1 can of creamed corn
- 1 can of green chilies
- 1 jalapeno pepper, minced
- 4 cups of vegetable broth
- 1 can of crushed tomatoes

Directions:
1. Put all the ingredients into the slow cooker.
2. Cook on low for four hours. Serve and enjoy.

Nutrition Value: Calories 145, Fat 2 g, Carbs 32g, Protein 4g

Delicious Special Veggie Stew

SmartPoints: 7

Servings: 8

Ingredients:

- ½ teaspoon of coriander
- 1 teaspoon of cumin
- 1 teaspoon of salt
- 1 can of lite coconut milk
- 1/3 cup of tomato paste
- ½ cup of chopped onion
- 2 tablespoons of grated ginger
- 7 cups of vegetable broth
- 2 carrots, diced
- 2 cups of red lentils

Directions:

1. Place all the ingredients in the crackpot.
2. Cook on low for about six hours.
3. Serve with yogurt.

Nutrition Value: Calories 236, Fat 4 g, Carbs 36g, Protein 14g

Healthy Mushroom Spinach Gnocchi Soup

Smart Points: 7

Servings: 6

Ingredients:
- 1 pack of gnocchi
- 4 cups of spinach
- 2 cups of sliced mushrooms
- 1 can of diced tomatoes
- ¼ cup of Italian seasoning
- ½ teaspoon of black pepper
- ½ teaspoon of salt
- 4 cups of chicken broth (low sodium)
- 2 celery ribs, chopped
- 2 carrots, chopped
- 1 onion, chopped
- 1 cup of parmesan cheese

Directions:
1. Place all the ingredients (except gnocchi, spinach, and cheese) in a slow cooker.
2. Cook on low for about five hours.
3. Add the gnocchi and spinach and cook for another hour.
4. Serve with parmesan cheese.

Nutrition Value: Calories 292, Fat 4 g, Carbs 43g, Protein 18g

Chapter 4: Slow Cooker Smart Points Chicken & Turkey Recipes

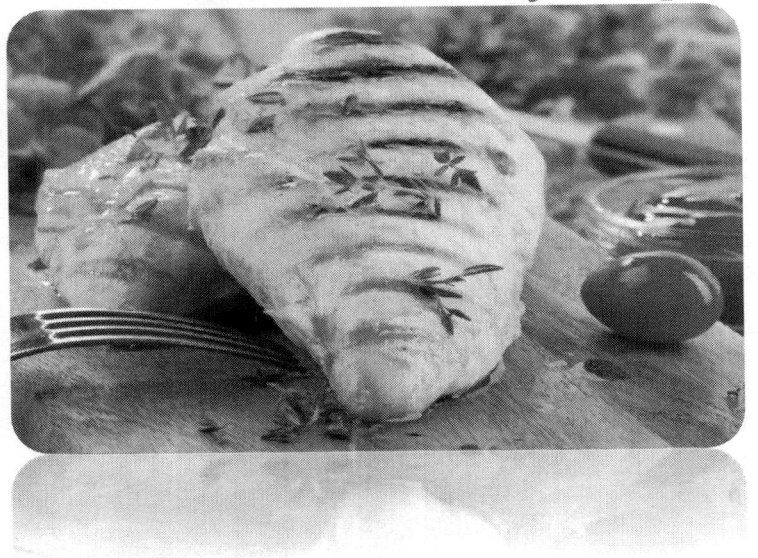

Lime Garlic Chicken

Serves: 4
SmartPoints: 7

Ingredients:
- 1 pound boneless, skinless chicken breast
- ½ teaspoon salt
- 1 teaspoon black pepper
- 1 cup chicken broth
- ½ cup fresh lime juice
- 1 tablespoon lime zest
- 4 cloves garlic, crushed and minced

- 1 tablespoon fresh tarragon, chopped
- 1 cup yellow onion, diced
- 1 habanero pepper, diced
- 3 cups cooked brown rice, for serving

Directions:

1. Season the chicken breasts with salt and black pepper.
2. In a blender, combine the chicken broth, fresh lime juice, lime zest, garlic, tarragon, onion, and habanero pepper. Blend until the mixture is smooth.
3. Pour the sauce over the chicken, and cover.
4. Cook on low for 6 hours.
5. Serve the chicken and sauce over cooked rice.

Nutrition Value: Calories 324, Fat 4 g, Carbs 37g, Protein 30g

Mushroom Cinnamon Chicken

Serves: 4

Smart Points: 6

Ingredients:
- 1 pound boneless, skinless chicken breasts
- ½ teaspoon salt
- 1 teaspoon black pepper
- 1 tablespoon olive oil
- 1 cup onion, thinly sliced
- 2 cloves garlic, crushed and minced
- 1 cup leeks, sliced thin
- ¼ cup dry white wine
- 1 tablespoon curry powder
- ½ teaspoon cinnamon
- 1 cup pearl barley
- 3 cups chicken stock
- 1 cup coconut milk
- 2 cups mushrooms, sliced

Directions:
1. Heat the olive oil in a skillet over medium heat.
2. Season the chicken breast with salt and black pepper.
3. Place the chicken breasts in the skillet and lightly brown on both sides. Transfer the chicken breasts to the slow cooker.
4. Next, add the onion, garlic, and leeks to the remaining oil in the skillet. Sauté the mixture for approximately 5 minutes.

5. Add in the white wine and continue cooking for 2-3 minutes while the wine reduces.
6. Stir in the curry powder and cinnamon. Add the vegetables from the skillet and the barley to the slow cooker with the chicken.
7. Pour in the chicken stock, cover and cook for 7 hours on low.
8. Remove the cover, and using two forks, shred the chicken.
9. Add in the coconut milk and the mushrooms.
10. Cover and cook an additional 45 minutes before serving.

Nutrition Value: Calories 270, Fat 7 g, Carbs 20g, Protein 29g

Brussels Sprouts Ginger Mustard Chicken

Serves: 6

SmartPoint: 5

Ingredients:
- 1 ½ pounds bone in chicken pieces, skin removed
- ½ teaspoon salt
- 1 teaspoon black pepper
- 2 teaspoons olive oil
- 2 cups Brussels sprouts, halved
- 2 cups sweet potatoes, peeled and cubed
- 1 ½ cups chicken broth
- ¼ cup red currant jelly
- ¼ cup fresh orange juice
- 1 tablespoon Dijon mustard
- 1 tablespoon apple cider vinegar
- 1 tablespoon fresh grated ginger

Directions:
1. Season the chicken with salt and black pepper.
2. Heat the olive oil in a skillet over medium heat. Add the chicken to the skillet and brown it evenly on all sides.
3. Remove the chicken from the skillet and place it in a slow cooker.
4. Add the Brussels sprouts and sweet potatoes to the slow cooker.

5. Next, combine the chicken broth, red currant jelly, fresh orange juice, Dijon mustard, apple cider vinegar, and fresh grated ginger in saucepan over medium low heat.

6. Cook, stirring frequently, until the jelly is dissolved and all of the ingredients are blended.

7. Remove the saucepan from the heat, let it cool slightly and then add it to the slow cooker.

8. Cover and cook for 8 hours on low heat.

Nutrition Value: Calories 198, Fat 5 g, Carbs 20g, Protein 19g

Tomato Mushroom Chicken

Smart Points: 4

Servings: 6

Ingredients:
- 1 cup of black olives
- ½ teaspoon of red pepper flakes
- 1 ½ teaspoon of capers, drained
- ½ cup of red wine
- 4 garlic cloves, sliced
- 1 pound of sliced mushrooms
- 1 green pepper, chopped
- 1 can of roasted tomatoes
- 4 tablespoons of tomato paste
- 2 diced celery stalks
- 1 onion, thinly sliced
- 2 pounds of boneless, skinless chicken breast (cut into chunks)

Directions:
1. Season the chicken with pepper and salt.
2. Add all the ingredients (except the black olives) in a slow cooker.
3. Cook on low for five hours.
4. Add the black olives and cook for another thirty minutes. Serve and enjoy.

Nutrition Value: Calories 246, Fat 4g, Carbs 14g, Protein 36g

Feta Olive Artichoke Chicken

SmartPoints: 3
Servings: 6

Ingredients:
- Salt
- Pepper
- 1 ½ cups of chicken broth (low sodium)
- 1 teaspoon of garlic powder
- 1 teaspoon of dried oregano
- 4 oz of feta cheese (reduced fat)
- 1 cup of chopped canned artichoke heart
- ¼ cup of sliced black olives
- ½ cup of chopped roasted red peppers
- 3 cups of finely-chopped spinach
- 2 pounds of skinless, boneless chicken breasts

Directions:
1. Mix the artichoke hearts, spinach, roasted red peppers, oregano, feta cheese, and garlic. Set aside.
2. Season the chicken breast with pepper and salt.
3. Using a knife, cut in the center of the chicken breasts to create a pocket.
4. Then, stuff the chicken breasts with the spinach mixture.
5. Place the chicken in the slow cooker. Cook for at least four hours.

Nutrition Value: Calories 222, Fat 7g, Carbs 8g, Protein 35g

Yummy Cumin Jalapeno Chicken

Smart Points: 6

Servings: 4

Ingredients:
- Pepper
- Salt
- 2 teaspoons of cumin
- 1 tablespoon of soy sauce
- 1/3 cup of chopped cilantro
- 1 onion, sliced
- 1 jalapeno pepper, chopped
- 2 poblano peppers
- ½ pound of tomatillos, quartered and husked
- 1 pound of boneless, skinless chicken thighs
- 1 pound of boneless, skinless chicken breasts

Directions:
1. Place the chicken in the slow cooker, then stir in the remaining ingredients.
2. Cook for four hours. Serve and enjoy.

Nutrition Value: Calories 204, Fat 4g, Carbs 8g, Protein 32g

Delicious Garlic Celery Buffalo Chicken

SmartPoints: 2
Servings: 6

Ingredients:

- ½ cup of buffalo hot sauce
- Pepper
- Salt
- 1 ½ cups of chicken broth (low sodium)
- 2 garlic cloves, sliced
- 1 onion, quartered
- 2 celery ribs, sliced
- 2 carrots, cubed
- 2 pounds of skinless, boneless chicken
- ½ cup of melted butter

Directions:

1. Place the chicken, salt, pepper, celery, garlic, carrots, onion, and broth in the slow cooker.
2. Cook on medium for four hours.
3. Remove from the slow cooker and drain the liquid. Shred the chicken.
4. Add the butter and the buffalo sauce.
5. Place the chicken mixture in a pan and heat for 15 minutes. Serve and enjoy.

Nutrition Value: Calories 165, Fat 2g, Carbs 5g, Protein 34g

Lemon Garlic Herbs Chicken

Servings: 4

Smart Points:7

Ingredients

- 2 cloves garlic, crushed
- 1 whole chicken
- 1 c. tablespoons dried oregano
- Pepper
- Salt
- 5 c. tablespoons water
- 2 c. tablespoons butter
- 4 c. tablespoon lemon juice
- 1 c. tablespoon of lemon zest

Directions:

1. Season chicken (inner part) with salt and pepper to taste.
2. Mix half of the oregano and garlic cloves. Rub the inside of the chicken with this mixture.
3. Melt butter in a skillet. Brown chicken on both sides. Then place it in the center of the slow cooker.
4. Sprinkle chicken with remaining oregano and the second garlic clove.
5. Add water to the pan to dissolve the chicken cooking residue. Then pour over chicken.
6. Cook the chicken at low temperature for 8 hours.
7. In the last hour of cooking, mix the lemon juice and zest. Pour over chicken.
8. When the chicken is cooked, remove from the crock pot and serve.
9. Degrease the chicken and serve as a sauce.

Nutrition Value: Calories 280, Fat 5g, Carbs 38g, Protein 12g

Italian Style Balsamic Chicken

Smart Points: 3
Servings: 6

Ingredients:
- Pepper
- Salt
- 6 cups of spinach
- 1 tablespoon of Italian seasoning
- 3 tablespoons of balsamic vinegar
- 4 garlic cloves, minced
- 1 sweet onion, sliced
- 28 oz canned tomatoes, drained
- 2 pounds of skinless, boneless chicken breasts

Directions:
1. Place the chicken in a slow cooker. Then, add pepper and salt. Stir in the balsamic vinegar, Italian seasoning, garlic, sweet onion, and canned tomatoes.
2. Cook for 30 minutes and then add the spinach.
3. Then, cook for another four hours. Serve and enjoy.

Nutrition Value: Calories 225, Fat 2g, Carbs 12g, Protein 34g

Delicious Mexican Style Casserole

Serves: 6

Smart Points: 5

Ingredients:
- 1 ½ pounds boneless, skinless chicken, cubed
- ½ teaspoon salt
- 1 teaspoon black pepper
- 1 teaspoon chili powder
- ½ teaspoon cumin
- ½ teaspoon cayenne powder
- 1 cup red onion, chopped
- 1 cup red bell pepper, chopped
- 1 cup poblano pepper, chopped
- 1 cup fresh corn kernels
- ½ cup canned green chilies
- 1 14 ounce can stewed tomatoes, with liquid
- ½ cup low sodium tomato juice
- 1 tablespoon cayenne pepper sauce
- ½ cup low fat sour cream
- ½ cup Monterey jack cheese, shredded

Directions:
1. Season the chicken with salt, black pepper, chili powder, cumin, and cayenne powder.
2. Add the red onion, red bell pepper, poblano pepper, corn kernels, and canned green chilies to the bottom of the slow cooker and stir.

3. Next, add the chicken on top of the vegetables followed by the stewed tomatoes and liquid.

4. Combine the cayenne pepper sauce with the tomato juice and add that to the slow cooker as well.

5. Cover and cook on low for 6 hours.

6. Remove the cover and stir in the low fat sour cream and Monterey jack cheese.

7. Cover and cook an additional 30 minutes before serving.

Nutrition Value: Calories 250, Fat 7g, Carbs 15g, Protein 34g

Tasty Savory Apple Chicken

Serves: 6

SmartPoints: 4

Ingredients:
- 1 ½ pounds bone in chicken pieces, skin removed
- 1 teaspoon salt
- 1 teaspoon black pepper
- 2 teaspoons olive oil
- 3 cups Granny Smith apples, peeled and sliced thick
- 1 tablespoon lemon juice
- 1 cup yellow onion, sliced
- 1 cup chicken broth
- 1 tablespoon fresh thyme, chopped
- 1 tablespoon fresh tarragon, chopped
- 2 cloves garlic, crushed and minced

Directions:
1. Season the chicken pieces with the salt and black pepper.
2. Add the olive oil to a large skillet over medium heat.
3. Place the chicken in the skillet and brown each piece lightly on all sides.
4. Place the apples in the slow cooker and sprinkle them with the lemon juice.
5. Combine the sliced onions with the apples and season the mixture with thyme, tarragon, and garlic.
6. Transfer the chicken from the skillet into the slow cooker and add in the chicken broth.
7. Cover and cook on low for 8 hours.

Nutrition Value: Calories 188, Fat 4g, Carbs 10g, Protein 26g

Simple Chili Chicken

Smart Points: 5
Servings: 6

Ingredients:
- Salt
- Pepper
- 1 tablespoon of lime juice
- 4 cups of chicken broth (low sodium)
- 1 teaspoon of oregano
- 2 tablespoons of cumin
- ½ cup of chopped cilantro
- 2 poblano peppers, diced
- 1 jalapeno, diced
- 4 garlic cloves, minced
- 1 onion, minced
- 1 can of white beans, drained
- 1.5 pounds of boneless, skinless chicken breast

Directions:
1. Place all the ingredients in the slow cooker and cook for four hours.
2. Remove the chicken from the slow cooker and shred.
3. Put back the shredded chicken and serve.

Nutrition Value: Calories: 278, Fat 3g, Carbs 30g, Protein 35g

Chicken Meatloaf

Serves: 8

SmartPoints: 7

Ingredients:
- 1 ½ pounds ground chicken
- ½ pound ground pork
- 2 egg whites
- 1 cup dry bread crumbs
- 4 cloves garlic, crushed and minced
- ½ cup canned green chilies
- 1 cup carrots, shredded
- 1 cup jarred salsa
- 1 teaspoon salt
- 1 teaspoon black pepper
- 1 teaspoon cumin
- 1 teaspoon smoked paprika

Directions:
1. Line your slow cooker with a slow cooker liner so that the meatloaf can easily be lifted out when it is ready to serve. You can also use a large loaf pan placed in your slow cooker with a bit of water around the bottom of the pan.
2. In a bowl, combine the ground chicken, ground pork, egg whites, and bread crumbs.
3. Next, add in the garlic, green chilies, carrots, and salsa.
4. Season the mixture with the salt, black pepper, cumin, and smoked paprika. Use your hands to blend the ingredients together.
5. Transfer the meat mixture to the lined slow cooker.

6. Press the meat mixture gently to spread it along the bottom.
7. Cover and cook on low for 8 hours.
8. Lift the foil out of the slow cooker to remove the meatloaf.
9. Let it sit several minutes before slicing and serving.

Nutrition Value: Calories: 263, Fat 12g, Carbs 15g, Protein 21g

Delicious Barbecue Turkey

Smart Points: 4

Servings: 8

Ingredients:
- ½ cup of chicken broth (low sodium)
- 1 cup of barbecue sauce
- ½ tablespoon of pepper
- 1 teaspoon of salt
- 2 garlic, mined
- 1 onion, sliced
- 2 apple, sliced
- ½ cup of applesauce
- 1 teaspoon of chili powder
- 1 teaspoon of cumin
- 2 pounds of boneless, skinless turkey breast

Directions:
1. Combine the cumin, applesauce, broth, salt, garlic, chili powder, pepper, and salt in a bowl. Set aside.
2. Place the onion, apples, and turkey in the slow cooker.
3. Pour the applesauce mixture on top of the turkey.
4. Cook on low for four hours.
5. Remove from heat and shred the turkey using two forks. Serve and enjoy.

Nutrition Value: Calories: 215, Fat 3g, Carbs 22g, Protein 25g

Pinto Beans Bay Leaf Turkey

Smart Points: 5

Servings: 8

Ingredients:

- ½ tablespoon of coriander
- ½ tablespoon of cumin
- 1 bay leaf
- 3 cups of chicken broth (low sodium)
- 1 can of pinto beans
- 1 can of hominy
- 1.5 pounds of skinless, boneless turkey
- 8 garlic cloves
- 1 onion, quartered
- 3 jalapeno peppers
- 2 poblano peppers
- 1 ½ pounds of husked tomatillos

Directions:

1. Preheat the oven to 500 degrees.
2. Place the onion, garlic cloves, jalapeno peppers, poblano peppers, and tomatillos on a baking sheet. Add a little bit of kosher salt. Then, roast for 15 minutes. Remove from the oven and let it cool for a few minutes.
3. Place the roasted garlic, peppers, and tomatillos in a blender. Process for one to three minutes and set aside.
4. Place the pinto beans, hominy, and bay leaf to the crackpot.
5. Add the turkey and pour the tomatillo mixture on top.
6. Cook on low for eight hours.
7. Add some garnish. Serve and enjoy.

Nutrition Value: Calories: 317, Fat 5g, Carbs 41g, Protein 29g

Cheesy Eggplant Eggplant Chicken

Serves: 6

Smart Points: 8

Ingredients:

- 1 pound ground chicken
- ½ teaspoon salt
- 1 teaspoon black pepper
- 1 large eggplant, peeled and cubed
- 1 cup onions, chopped
- 2 cloves garlic, crushed and minced
- 2 teaspoons olive oil
- 2 cups tomatoes, chopped
- 1 cup bulgur
- 3 cups chicken broth
- ½ cup fresh parsley, chopped
- ¼ cup fresh mint, chopped
- ½ cup feta cheese, crumbled

Directions:

1. Season the ground chicken with the salt and black pepper, and then place it in the bottom of the slow cooker.
2. Heat the olive oil over medium heat in a large skillet.
3. Add the eggplant, onion, and garlic to the skillet and sauté the vegetable mixture for approximately 3-5 minutes.
4. Transfer the vegetables from the skillet to the slow cooker. Add in the bulgur, chopped tomatoes, and the chicken broth. Cover and cook on low for 6 hours.
7. Remove the cover and stir in the parsley, mint, and feta cheese. Cover and let sit for 15 minutes before serving.

Nutrition Value: Calories: 302, Fat 12g, Carbs 28g, Protein 20g

Yummy Curry Chicken

Smart Points: 5

Servings: 6

Ingredients:
- ½ teaspoon of cinnamon
- ½ teaspoon of pepper
- 1 teaspoon of salt
- 1 teaspoon of cumin
- 1 teaspoon of turmeric
- ¼ cup of limes
- 3 garlic cloves
- 1 jalapeno pepper, chopped
- 1 ginger, chopped
- 2 cups of basil
- 1 can of coconut milk
- 2 pounds of boneless, skinless chicken

Directions:
1. Place the ginger, basil, coconut milk, turmeric, lime juice, curry powder, pepper, salt, and cinnamon in a blender. Process for a minute or two. Set aside.
2. Place the chicken in the slow cooker. Then, pour the sauce over the top.
3. Cook for four hours. Serve and enjoy.

Nutrition Value: Calories: 226, Fat 4g, Carbs 4g, Protein 33g

Chapter 5: Slow Cooker Smart points Beef &Pork Recipes

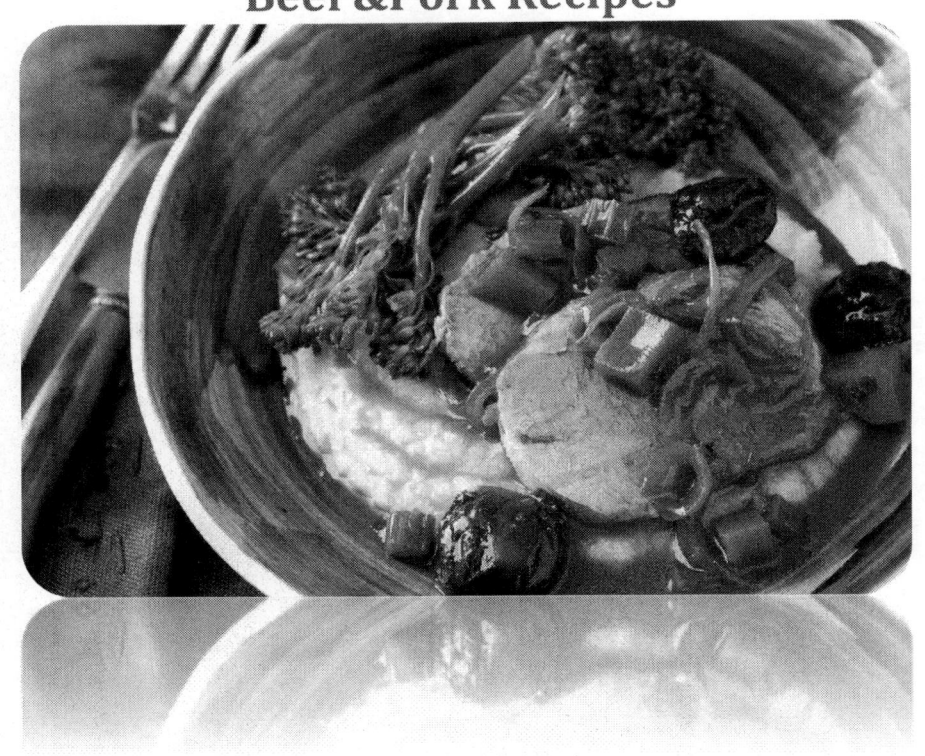

Yummy Pulled Pork

Servings: 6

Smart Points: 5

Ingredients:
- 2 lb. roast pork shoulder
- salt and pepper
- 1/2 cup ketchup
- 1/2 cup brown sugar
- 1/3 cup red wine vinegar

Directions:
1. Preheat the slow cooker to low power for 15 minutes
2. Add salt and pepper to the roast pork and place in slow cooker. Mix the ketchup, brown sugar and vinegar in a bowl. Pour meat in the over.
3. Cook for 8 hours on low heat.
4. Transfer roast to a platter and cut into 3 or four large pieces.
5. Shred meat with two forks and put in the slow cooker for 1 hour.

Nutrition Value: Calories: 197, Fat 12g, Carbs 1g, Protein 20g

Garlic Worcestershire Sauce Braised Beef

Smart Points: 3
Servings: 6

Ingredients:
- ¼ teaspoon of coriander
- ¼ teaspoon of oregano
- ½ teaspoon of cumin
- 2 tablespoons of lime juice
- 1 tablespoon of Worcestershire sauce
- 1 cup of canned tomatoes
- ¼ cup of beef broth (low sodium)
- 2 jalapeno peppers
- 2 garlic cloves, sliced
- 1 red bell pepper, diced
- 1 sweet onion, diced
- 2 pounds of lean beef eye round

Directions:
1. Season the beef with salt and pepper and then place in a slow cooker.
2. Add the peppers, onion, and garlic.
3. In a bowl, combine the tomatoes, beef broth, lime juice, Worcestershire sauce, cumin, lime juice, coriander, and oregano. Then, pour the mixture over the beef.
4. Cook on low for about eight hours. Serve and enjoy.

Nutrition Value: Calories: 233, Fat 5g, Carbs 8g, Protein 36g

Beef Taco Filling

Smart Points: 3
Servings: 6

Ingredients:
- Pepper
- Salt
- 3 pounds of lean top round roast
- ½ teaspoon of cumin
- ½ teaspoon of coriander
- 1 teaspoon of oregano
- 4 tablespoons of chipotle chilies in adobo sauce
- 1 onion, sliced
- 4 cloves of garlic
- 2 dried guajillo chili peppers
- 2 dried ancho chili peppers
- 2 cups of chicken broth (low sodium)

Directions:
1. Combine the chicken broth and peppers in a large bowl and let sit for about 30 minutes.
2. Then place the chicken broth mixture in a blender. Add the onion, garlic, oregano, chipotles, cumin, and coriander. Blend for a minute or two.
3. Season the beef with pepper and salt, then place in the slow cooker.
4. Pour the chicken broth sauce over the beef.
5. Cook on low for about eight hours.
6. Shred and place on top of tacos.

Nutrition Value: Calories: 237, Fat 7g, Carbs 8g, Protein 43g

Thyme Ginger Apricots Pork Chops

Serves: 6

Smart Points : 10

Ingredients:
- 1 ½ pounds boneless pork chops
- 2 teaspoons olive oil
- ½ teaspoon salt
- ½ teaspoon black pepper
- 1 teaspoon thyme
- ½ teaspoon ground ginger
- 1 cup red onion, sliced
- 1 cups dried apricot halves
- ½ cup dried cranberries
- 1 cup unsweetened apple juice
- 2 cups sweet potatoes, peeled and cubed

Directions:
1. Brush the pork chops with olive oil and season them with salt, black pepper, thyme, and ground ginger.
2. Heat a skillet over medium heat.
3. Place the pork chops in the skillet and brown lightly on both sides.
4. Transfer the pork chops to the slow cooker.
5. To the slow cooker, add in the red onion, dried apricot halves, dried cranberries, unsweetened apple juice, and sweet potatoes.
6. Cover and cook on low for 6 hours.

Nutrition Value: Calories: 300, Fat 7g, Carbs 37g, Protein 23g

Yummy Chili Taco Filling

Serves: 6

Smart Points: 7

Ingredients:

- 1 pound lean ground beef
- 1 teaspoon salt
- 1 teaspoon black pepper
- 1 teaspoon ground cumin
- 1 teaspoon chili powder
- ½ teaspoon cayenne powder
- 1 teaspoon garlic powder
- 1 teaspoon paprika
- ½ teaspoon cinnamon
- 1 tablespoon tomato paste
- 1 tablespoon lime juice
- ¾ cup beef broth
- 1 cup onion, diced
- 2 cloves garlic, crushed and minced
- 1 cup red bell pepper, diced
- 1 cup poblano pepper, diced
- 1 tablespoon jalapeno pepper, diced
- ¼ cup chipotle pepper in adobo sauce, chopped
- ¼ cup fresh cilantro, chopped

Directions:

1. Place the ground beef in the slow cooker and season it with the salt, black pepper, ground cumin, chili powder, cayenne powder, garlic powder, paprika, and cinnamon. Mix well.

2. Next, add in the tomato paste, lime juice, and beef broth and mix well.

3. Finally, add in the onion, garlic, red bell pepper, poblano pepper, jalapeno pepper, chipotle pepper with the adobo sauce, and the fresh cilantro. Lightly mix.

4. Cover and cook on low for 8 hours.

5. Serve on lettuce leaves or tortillas with your favorite taco garnishes.

Nutrition Value: Calories: 225, Fat 15g, Carbs 6g, Protein 15g

Tasty Mushroom Pork Meatloaf

Serves: 10

Smart Points: 10

Ingredients:

- 1 ½ pounds lean ground beef
- ½ pound ground pork
- 2 egg whites
- 2 cups portobello mushrooms, chopped
- ¼ cup shallots, diced
- 2 cloves garlic, crushed and minced
- 1 cup seasoned bread crumbs
- 1 cup fresh parsley, chopped
- 2 tablespoons Worcestershire sauce
- 1 teaspoon salt
- 1 teaspoon black pepper
- ¼ cup fresh basil, chopped
- ¼ pound prosciutto

Directions:

1. Line your slow cooker with a slower cooker liner so that the meatloaf can easily be lifted out when ready to serve.
2. In a bowl, combine the lean ground beef, the ground pork, and the egg whites.
3. Next, add in the portobello mushrooms, shallots, garlic, seasoned bread crumbs, and parsley.
4. Season the meat mixture with the Worcestershire sauce, salt, black pepper, and basil. Mix gently with your hands until all of the ingredients are incorporated throughout.

5. Place the meatloaf mixture in the slow cooker and gently press down until the meatloaf evenly covers the bottom.
6. Place pieces of prosciutto over the meatloaf.
7. Cover and cook on low for 8 hours.
8. Remove the meatloaf by lifting out the liner, and let it rest for at least 10 minutes before serving.

Nutrition Value: Calories: 323, Fat 20g, Carbs 6g, Protein 24g

Mustard Chili Garlic Beef Ribs

Serves: 8

Smart Points: 5

Ingredients:

- 2 pounds beef ribs, extra fat removed
- 1 cup onion, chopped
- 2 cloves garlic, chopped
- ¼ cup lemon juice
- ¼ cup Dijon mustard
- 1 tablespoon tomato paste
- ¼ cup Worcestershire sauce
- 1 teaspoon salt
- 1 teaspoon chili powder
- 1 teaspoon brown sugar
- ½ cup beef broth or water

Directions:

1. In a blender, combine the onion, garlic, lemon juice, Dijon mustard, tomato paste, and Worcestershire sauce.
2. Season the beef ribs with the salt, chili powder, and brown sugar.
3. Liberally brush the mixture from the blender over the surface of the ribs.
4. Pour the beef broth or the water into the bottom of a slow cooker.
5. Place the ribs in the slow cooker, and add in any remaining sauce from the blender.
6. Cover and cook on low for 10 hours.

Nutrition Value: Calories: 192, Fat 8g, Carbs 4g, Protein 23g

Cashew Coconut Tenderloin

Serves: 8

Smart Points : 6

Ingredients:

- 2 pounds pork tenderloin
- 2 teaspoons olive oil
- ½ teaspoon salt
- 1 teaspoon black pepper
- ½ cup coconut milk
- ½ cup chicken broth
- ¼ cup low sodium soy sauce
- 1 tablespoon brown sugar
- ¼ cup no sugar added cashew butter
- 1 tablespoon crushed red pepper flakes
- ¼ cup chopped cashews for garnish (optional)

Directions:

1. Brush the pork tenderloin with olive oil and season it with the salt and black pepper.
2. Place the tenderloin in a skillet over medium heat and cook it just until lightly browned on all sides.
3. Transfer the tenderloin to the slow cooker.
4. In a bowl, whisk together the coconut milk, chicken broth, low sodium soy sauce, brown sugar, cashew butter, and crushed red pepper flakes.
5. Pour the sauce over the pork tenderloin.
6. Cover and cook on low for 8 hours.
7. Remove the tenderloin from the slow cooker and let it rest for at least ten minutes before slicing.
8. Serve garnished with chopped cashews, if desired.

Nutrition Value: Calories: 282, Fat 12g, Carbs 4g, Protein 33g

Jalapeno Ginger Beef in Sauce

Smart Points: 5

Servings: 8

Ingredients:
- 2 tablespoons of seasoned rice wine vinegar
- 1 tablespoon of grated ginger
- 2 jalapeno peppers, diced
- ½ red onion, diced
- 10 garlic cloves
- 1/3 cup of soy sauce (low sodium)
- ½ cup of brown sugar
- 2.5 pounds of lean round roast

Directions:
1. In a small bowl, combine the soy sauce, sugar, jalapeno pepper, red onion, sesame seeds, and rice vinegar. Set aside.
2. Place the garlic and the beef in a slow cooker and pour the rice vinegar over them.
3. Cook on low for nine hours.
4. Shred the beef and cook for another 30 minutes.
5. Serve over tortilla or pasta.

Nutrition Value: Calories: 256, Fat 5g, Carbs 17g, Protein 37g

Yummy Shredded Beef

Serves: 10
Smart Points: 8

Ingredients:
- 2 pounds lean beef roast, excess fat trimmed
- 1 tablespoon olive oil
- ½ teaspoon salt
- 1 teaspoon coarse ground black pepper
- ¼ cup tomato paste
- 1 cup vegetable juice
- 1 cup tomatoes, chopped
- 1 tablespoon honey
- 1 cup onion, chopped
- 4 cloves garlic, chopped
- 1 teaspoon crushed red pepper flakes
- 2 teaspoons ground cumin
- ¼ cup unsweetened cocoa powder
- 1 teaspoon cinnamon
- 2 teaspoons Mexican oregano
- 2 tablespoons cornmeal

Directions:
1. Brush the roast with the olive oil and season it with the salt and coarse ground black pepper.
2. Heat a skillet over medium heat.
3. Add the roast to the skillet and brown lightly on all sides. Transfer the roast to a slow cooker.

4. In a blender, combine the tomato paste, vegetable juice, tomatoes, honey, onion, garlic, crushed red pepper flakes, ground cumin, unsweetened cocoa powder, cinnamon, Mexican oregano, and the cornmeal. Blend until well combined.

5. Pour the mixture over the roast, and use a basting brush to evenly coat all sides of the meat.

6. Cover and cook on low for 8 hours.

7. Remove the cover and let the roast rest for 15 minutes.

8. Shred the beef and toss it with any sauce that is remaining in the bottom of the slow cooker.

9. Serve the shredded beef on a bed of salad greens or your favorite sandwich roll.

Nutrition Value: Calories: 322, Fat 18g, Carbs 9g, Protein 27g

Delight Roast Beef

Servings: 8

Smart Points: 1

Ingredients:
- 2 lb. roast beef
- 1 c. tablespoon salt
- 1 c. tablespoons ground black pepper
- 2 c. in dried parsley tea
- 2 c. dried oregano tea
- 4 potatoes, chopped
- 2 cups baby carrots
- 1 tomato, chopped
- 1/2 yellow onion, chopped
- 1 can (213 ml) tomato sauce
- 1/2 cup water

Directions:
1. Sprinkle salt roast, pepper, parsley and oregano on roast beef. Place in slow cooker and add the potato chunks, carrots, tomatoes and onion.
2. Pour the tomato sauce and water on top.
3. Cover and cook on high (HIGH) for 4 hours.

Nutrition Value: Calories: 56, Fat 3.64g, Carbs 0g, Protein 6g

Onion Chili Beef Roast Tacos

Smart Points: 3
Servings: 8

Ingredients:
- 1 cup of beef broth
- 1 bay leaf
- 1 onion, chopped
- 2 pounds of lean tri-tip roast
- 1 teaspoon of black pepper
- 1 teaspoon of salt
- 1 tablespoon of ancho chili powder
- 1 tablespoon of smoked paprika
- 8 garlic cloves

Directions:
1. Place the garlic in a food processor and process until smooth.
2. In a bowl, combine the garlic paste, salt, pepper, paprika, and chili powder.
3. Rub the garlic mixture on the tri-tip roast.
4. Place the onion and beef broth in the crackpot. Add the tri-tip on top and cook on low for about eight hours.
5. Shred the meat and cook for another 30 minutes.
6. Serve with warm tortillas or lettuce wrap.

Nutrition Value: Calories: 196, Fat 8g, Carbs 4g, Protein 25g

Delicious Stuffed Flank Roll

Serves: 8

Smart Points: 6

Ingredients:
- 2 pound flank steak
- ½ teaspoon salt
- 1 teaspoon black pepper
- 1 tablespoon olive oil
- ¼ cup shallots
- 2 cloves garlic, crushed and minced
- ¼ cup pistachios, chopped
- 1 cup mushrooms, chopped
- ½ cup seasoned bread crumbs
- ¼ cup fresh parsley, chopped
- 1 egg white
- ½ cup beef stock
- ¼ cup Worcestershire sauce
- ¼ cup dry red wine

Directions:
1. Trim off any excess fat from the flank steak and season it with salt and black pepper.
2. Place the olive oil in a skillet over medium heat.
3. Add the shallots and garlic, to the skillet and sauté for 1-2 minutes.
4. Next, add in the pistachios and the mushrooms and cook, stirring frequently for 2-3 minutes.

5. Remove the skillet from the heat and let it cool slightly.
6. To the vegetables in the skillet, add in the seasoned bread crumbs, parsley, and egg white. Use a fork to combine the ingredients.
7. Spread the pistachio mushroom mixture over the surface of the flank steak.
8. Roll the flank steak widthwise, similar to how you would roll a jelly roll.
9. Secure the roll with kitchen twine or wooden toothpicks.
10. Place the roll in the slow cooker.
11. Add the beef stock, Worcestershire sauce, and dry red wine to the slow cooker.
12. Cover and cook on low for 8 hours.
13. Remove the roll from the slow cooker and let it rest for 15 minutes before slicing. Remove twine and/or toothpicks before serving.

Nutrition Value: Calories: 257, Fat 12g, Carbs 8g, Protein 26g

Champagne Slow Cooker Sauerbraten

Serves: 10
Smart Points: 6

Ingredients:
- 2 pound boneless beef roast
- ½ teaspoon salt
- 1 teaspoon black pepper
- 2 teaspoons olive oil
- 1 cup onion, sliced
- 2 cloves garlic, crushed and minced
- 1 tablespoon flour
- 1 cup champagne vinegar
- 1 cup beef broth
- ¼ cup sugar
- 1 bay leaf
- 1 tablespoon peppercorns
- 3-4 whole cloves
- ½ cup low fat sour cream

Directions:
1. Season the beef roast with salt and black pepper and then place it in the slow cooker.
2. Heat the olive oil in a deep skillet over medium heat.
3. Add the onion and garlic to the skillet and sauté for 1-2 minutes before sprinkling them with flour. Stir and cook for 1-2 minutes more.

4. Next, add in the champagne vinegar, beef broth, sugar, bay leaf, peppercorns, and cloves.

5. Bring the liquid to a boil and continue boiling for 1 minute. Remove the skillet from the stove and let it cool slightly.

6. Pour the sauce into the slow cooker.

7. Cover and cook on low for 8 hours.

8. Remove the roast from the slow cooker and set it aside to rest for at least 15 minutes.

9. Stir the sour cream into the sauce remaining in the slow cooker.

10. Slice the roast and serve it with sauce.

Nutrition Value: Calories: 324, Fat 18g, Carbs 7g, Protein 26g

Delicious Coconut Curry Beef

Smart Points: 4

Servings: 4

Ingredients:
- 2 teaspoons of lime juice
- ½ cup of light coconut milk
- 1 tablespoon of soy sauce
- 1 teaspoon of lime zest
- 1 ½ cups of canned tomato sauce
- 1 tablespoons of red curry paste
- 1 teaspoon of grated ginger
- 2 garlic cloves, minced
- 1 leek, sliced
- 1 pound lean ground beef

Directions:
1. In a pan, brown the beef for around five to ten minutes over medium heat.
2. Remove the beef from the pan and then place it in a crackpot.
3. Add the garlic, leek, red curry paste, ginger, lime zest, tomato sauce, and soy sauce.
4. Cook on low for about four hours.
5. Open the lid and add the lime juice and coconut milk.
6. Cook for another fifteen minutes. Serve and enjoy.

Nutrition Value: Calories: 213, Fat 8g, Carbs 10g, Protein 26g

Tasty Beef Stew

Servings: 4

Smart Points: 5

Ingredients:
- 2 lb. beef cubes
- 1/4 cup all-purpose flour
- 1 c. paprika
- 1/2 c. pepper tea
- 1 bay leaf
- 1 garlic clove
- 3 diced potatoes
- 1 foot sliced celery
- 2 onions, chopped
- 1 c. Tea soy sauce
- 375ml beef stock

Directions:
1. In a bowl, mix flour, paprika, and pepper.
2. Coat beef cubes.
3. Place the beef in a slow cooker. Add the rest of the INGREDIENTS and mix well.
4. Cook at for 4-6 hours at high temperature for or low temperature of 10 to 12 hours.

Nutrition Value: Calories: 207, Fat 6g, Carbs 22g, Protein 17g

Spicy Oregano Pulled Pork

Smart Points: 3

Servings: 6

Ingredients:

- 1 tablespoon of apple cider vinegar
- 1 cup of chicken broth
- 4 garlic cloves, minced
- 1 onion, diced
- 2 pounds of lean pork tenderloin
- ¼ teaspoon of coriander
- ¼ teaspoon of cinnamon
- ½ teaspoon of pepper
- 1 tablespoon of oregano
- 1 teaspoon of ground cumin
- 1 teaspoon of salt
- 1 teaspoon of chili powder
- 1 tablespoon of paprika

Directions:

1. Mix all the spices together and rub over pork.
2. Then, place the pork in the crockpot. Add the onions and chicken broth.
3. Cook for five hours on low.
4. Remove from the crackpot and shred.
5. If you want to make the pork crispy, broil the shredded pork for three minutes. Serve and enjoy.

Nutrition Value: Calories: 190, Fat 4g, Carbs 5g, Protein 3g

Spicy Tumeric Honey Pork Chops

Smart Points: 3

Servings: 4

Ingredients:

- ¼ cup of soy sauce (low sodium)
- ¼ cup of chili sauce
- 1 cup of minced onions
- ¼ cup honey
- 1 teaspoon of turmeric powder
- 1 pound of pork chops (lean)

Directions:

1. In a bowl, combine all the ingredients. Mix well.
2. Put everything in a slow cooker. Cook for five hours on low.
3. Check if meat is tender. Serve right away.

Nutrition Value: Calories: 212, Fat 4g, Carbs 12g, Protein 31g

Apple Pork Tenderloin

Smart Points: 3

Servings: 6

Ingredients:
- ½ teaspoon of black pepper
- 1 ½ teaspoon of kosher salt
- 2 tablespoon of whole grain mustard
- 2 apples, sliced
- 1 onion, sliced thinly
- 2 pounds of lean tenderloin

Directions:
1. Season the pork with pepper and salt. Then, place it in a slow cooker.
2. Spread the honey and mustard on the pork.
3. Cover the pork with apples and onions.
4. Cook for around six hours.
5. Remove from the slow cooker. Slice and serve.

Nutrition Value: Calories: 232, Fat 4g, Carbs 17g, Protein 31g

6. Place the browned tenderloin on top of the spinach mixture.
7. Cover and cook on low for 8 hours.
8. Remove the pork tenderloin from the slow cooker and let it rest for 10 minutes.
9. While the tenderloin is resting, add the low fat sour cream and parmesan cheese to the spinach mixture.
10. Cover and cook until heated through.
11. Slice the tenderloin and serve with the Florentine sauce.

Nutrition Value: Calories: 281, Fat 8g, Carbs 3g, Protein 37g

Sesame Ginger Onion Pork

Smart Points: 5

Servings: 8

Ingredients:
- 2 tablespoons of sesame seeds
- 1 tablespoon of rice wine vinegar
- 2 tablespoons of grated ginger root
- 2 jalapenos, diced
- ½ cup of diced red onion
- 10 whole garlic cloves
- 1/3 cup of soy sauce (low sodium)
- ½ cup of brown sugar
- 3 pounds of pork tenderloin

Directions:
1. Combine the soy sauce, sugar, onion, ginger, jalapeno pepper, sesame seeds, and rice vinegar in a small bowl.
2. Add the pork in a slow cooker.
3. Cook on low for eight hours.
4. Shred the pork and serve.

Nutrition Value: Calories: 268, Fat 5g, Carbs18g, Protein 37g

Garlic Sweet and Sour Pork

Serves: 6

Smart Points: 10

Ingredients:

- 1 ½ pounds pork loin, cut into cubes
- ½ teaspoon salt
- 1 teaspoon black pepper
- 1 tablespoon corn starch
- ½ cup soy sauce
- ¼ cup brown sugar
- ¼ cup chicken broth
- ¼ cup apple cider vinegar
- 1 tablespoon ketchup
- 2 cloves garlic, crushed and minced
- ½ cup onion, diced
- 1 cup red bell peppers, sliced thick
- 1 cup green bell peppers, sliced thick
- 4 cups cooked brown rice for serving

Directions:

1. Begin by seasoning the pork with the salt and black pepper. Sprinkle the cornstarch onto the pork and toss the pieces to evenly coat them. Place the cubed pork in the bottom of the slow cooker.

2. Next, combine the soy sauce, brown sugar, chicken broth, apple cider vinegar, ketchup, and garlic in a separate bowl. Whisk together until well combined and then pour the contents over the pork. Add the onions, red bell pepper, and green bell pepper to the slow cooker. Cover and cook on low for 6 hours. Serve with cooked brown rice.

Nutrition Value: Calories: 440, Fat 12g, Carbs 45g, Protein 35g

Chapter 6: Slow Cooker Smart Points Vegetarian Recipes

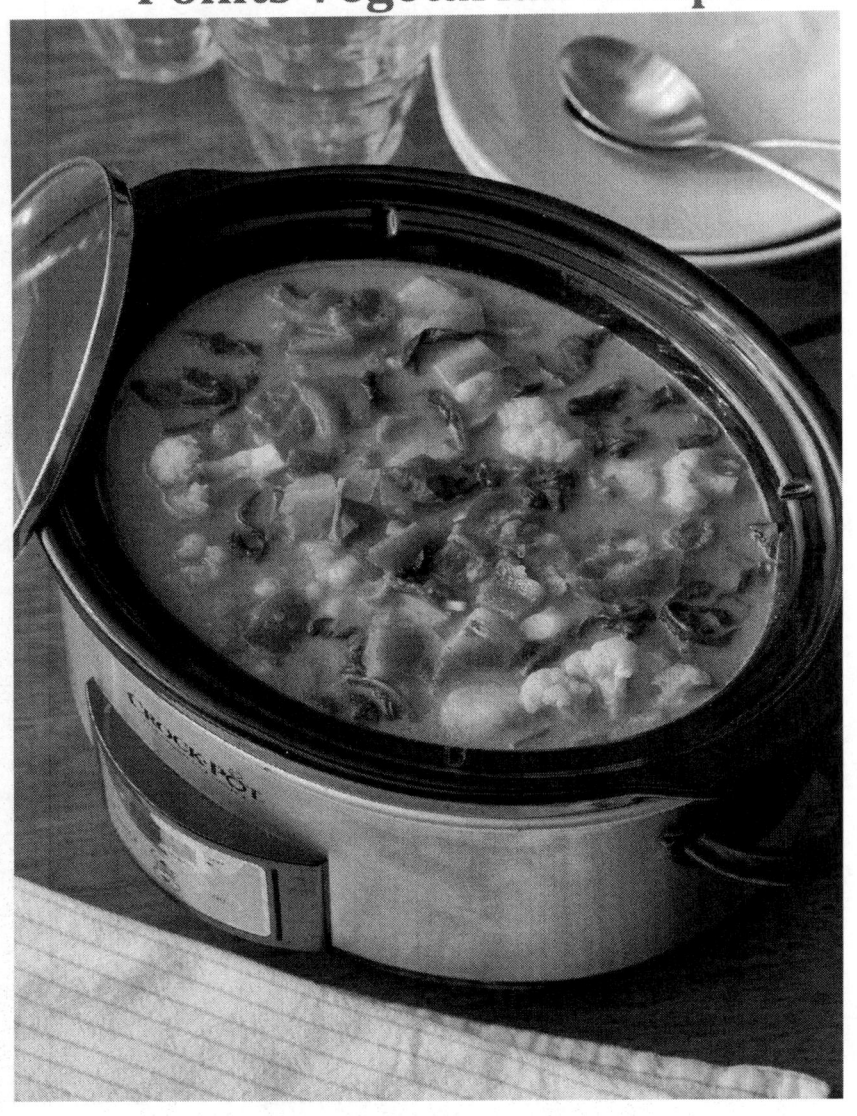

Yummy Black Bean Enchiladas with Spinach

Serve: 8

Smart Points: 7

Ingredients:
- Ground black pepper (to taste)
- Sea salt (to taste)
- Lime juice (1 lime)
- Chili powder (1 tsp.)
- Coriander (1 tsp. ground)
- Cumin (1 tsp. ground)
- Sharp cheddar cheese (1.5 cups shredded)
- Sour cream (.5 cups)
- Salsa Verde (24 oz.)
- Whole wheat tortilla (8)
- Corn (1 cup)
- Black beans (15 oz. rinsed, drained)
- Spinach (16 oz. frozen, thawed, squeezed)

Directions:
- Place half the total number of black beans in a large bowl and mash them prior to adding in the pepper, salt, lime juice, chili powder, coriander, cumin, other black beans, corn and spinach and mix well.

- Add half of the salsa to the slow cooker before adding the bean mixture to each tortilla and rolling tightly. Ideally all of the rolled tortillas will fit in a single layer in the slow cooker.
- Add in the rest of the salsa along with the cheese and let everything cook, covered, on a low setting for 3 hours.
- Top with jalapenos, onions, cilantro and sour cream prior to serving.

Nutrition Value: Calories: 217, Fat 3g, Carbs 30g, Protein 26g

Delicious Vegetable Fusion

Servings: 12

Points: 2

Ingredients:
- Olive oil
- 1 onion
- 4 carrots
- 4 stalks celery
- 1 turnip
- 1 can (700 mL) diced tomatoes
- 1 can tomato soup
- 8 cups chicken broth
- Fresh parsley
- Celery leaves
- Salt to taste
- Pepper

Ingredients:
1. Chop and fry the onion in a pan with olive oil. Add onion in slow cooker.
2. Cut the vegetables. Add all INGREDIENTS and vegetables in slow cooker. Simmer on low for 6 hours or on high for 3 hours.

Nutrition Value: Calories: 64, Fat 0g, Carbs 14g, Protein 2g

Tasty Polenta and Beans

Servings: 4

Smart Points: 8

Ingredients:

- 1 tsp. fresh parsley
- 1 tsp. fresh sage
- 2 garlic cloves, minced
- 1 can rinsed cannellini beans
- 4 cups of water
- 1/2 tsp. salt
- 2 tbsps. olive oil
- 1 cup yellow dry polenta
- 1/4 tsp. ground pepper
- 1 can diced tomatoes

Directions:

1. In a slow cooker, heat olive oil. Add garlic and parsley and cook for 60 seconds.
2. Add tomatoes and sage and cook until all liquid evaporates. That could mean 10 minutes.
3. Add beans, black pepper, and 1/8 teaspoon salt. Reduce the heat and cover. While stirring, cook for 30 minutes.
4. Add ½ teaspoon salt and 4 cups of water as you stir. Cook for 45 minutes while keeping it covered.
5. Get off the cover and cook for a maximum of 10 minutes. Cover again and cook for around 15 minutes then get it uncovered again and cook for two minutes as you constantly stir. You can now serve you polenta preferably with bean mixture.

Nutrition Value: Calories: 284, Fat 2g, Carbs 48g, Protein 11.1g

Garlic Vegan Chili

Servings: 6

Points: 6

Ingredients:

- 1 onion, finely chopped
- 2 garlic cloves, finely chopped
- 1 cup frozen corn kernels
- 2 carrots, peeled and diced
- 1 1/2 green bell pepper, diced
- 2 stalks celery, diced
- 2 packages Veggie Ground (original) Yves Veggie
- 1 can red kidney beans drained and rinsed
- 1 can black beans, drained and rinsed
- 1 can diced tomatoes
- 1 tomato saucebox
- 1 c. Tea chili
- 1 c. with dried oregano
- 1 c. Tea ground cumin
- Salt and pepper to taste
- Basmati rice to accompany

Directions:

1. Add the first 11 INGREDIENTS in slow cooker. Add chili powder, oregano, and cumin. Add salt and pepper and mix lightly.
2. Cover and cook on low for 6-8 hours or on high heat for 4 hours.
3. Serve with basmati rice if desired.

Nutrition Value: Calories: 229, Fat 2g, Carbs 48g, Protein 6g

Squash Soup

Serve: 12

Smart Points: 5

Ingredients:
- Water (2 cups)
- Vegetable broth (6 cups)
- Salt (1.25 tsp.)
- Cinnamon (2 sticks)
- Ginger (1 T minced)
- Brown Sugar (2 T)
- Onions (2 sliced)
- Olive oil (2 T)
- Butternut squash (6 lbs. sliced)

Directions:
- Start by making sure your oven is heated to 350 degrees F.
- Place the squash halves onto a baking sheet before placing the sheet in the oven and letting it cook 15 minutes. After it has finished baking, remove it from the stove to allow it to cool.
- As the squash cools, place a pan on the oven over a medium/high heat add in the oil and the onion and let it cook for 3 minutes before adding in the garlic, ginger and brown sugar and letting everything cook for an additional minute.
- Add the results to a slow cooker and let them cook, covered, on a low setting for 6 hours.
- Once the ingredients are done cooking, discard the cinnamon sticks and add everything else to a blender and blend well prior to serving.

Nutrition Value: Calories: 131, Fat 2g, Carbs 28g, Protein 4g

Shallots Pumpkin Braised Stew

Servings: 8

Smart Points: 6

Ingredients:

- 2 c. table olive oil
- 3 cups quartered French shallots 6 cloves of garlic
- 1/2 c. makers dried sage
- 4 t squash cubed
- 3 cups vegetable broth
- 1/2 cup dry white wine
- 1/4 c. Salt
- 1/4 c. black pepper tea mill
- 1 can kidney beans, rinsed and drained
- 1 can of white beans, rinsed and drained
- 2 c. flour
- Water 1/3 cup
- 1/4 cup fresh parsley, chopped

Directions:

1. In a skillet, heat oil and add shallots, garlic, and sage and cook for 7 minutes or until the shallots and garlic are golden. Put the shallot mixture in slow cooker.
2. Add squash, broth, wine, salt, pepper, and red beans. Put the beans in a bowl, mash with a potato masher, and then add to the simmering use.
3. Cover and cook on low for 4 hours.
4. In a bowl, mix flour and water. Add flour mixture and parsley in the slow cooker and mix. Cover and cook on high for 15 minutes or until sauce is thickened.

Nutrition Value: Calories: 221, Fat 9g, Carbs 31g, Protein 6g

Onion Split Pea Soup

Serve: 12

Smart Points: 2

Ingredients:
- Carrot (1 cup chopped)
- Garlic (1 T minced)
- Onion (.5 cups chopped fine)
- Vegetable broth (8 cups)
- Split peas (16 oz. dried)

Directions:
- Add all of the ingredients to a slow cooker and let them cook, covered, on a high setting for 6 hours.
- Once the ingredients are done cooking add everything else to a blender and blend well prior to serving.

Nutrition Value: Calories: 85, Fat 2g, Carbs 7.7g, Protein 8.3g

Slow Cooker Stuffed Peppers

Servings: 6

Smart Points: 6

Ingredients:
- 3 c. table olive oil (45 ml)
- 1/3 cup pine nuts or almonds sticks
- 1 chopped onion
- 2 garlic cloves, finely chopped
- Parboiled rice 1 cup (250 ml)
- 1/4 cup currants or raisins (60 ml)
- 2 c. in dried dill (30 ml)
- 2 c. with dried mint (30 ml)
- 1/ 4 c. salt tea (6 mL)
- 1 c. makers sugar (5 mL)
- 3/4 c. Tea ground cinnamon (4 ml)
- 1/2 c. Tea brewed spice of Jamaica (2 ml)
- 1/4 c. black pepper tea mill (1 ml)
- 2 cups boiling water (500 ml)
- 1 diced zucchini
- 6 peppers
- Water 1/2 cup (125 ml)
- 2 c. lemon juice (30 ml)
- 2 c. table fresh parsley, chopped (30 ml)

Directions:
1. Heat 2 tbsp. of oil in a medium sized saucepan over medium heat.

2.   Add the pine nuts and cook, stirring, for about 2 minutes or until lightly browned.

3.   Add garlic and onion and cook while occasionally stirring for 2 minutes. Add rice, currants, dill, mint, salt, sugar, cinnamon, allspice and pepper and to boiling water.

4.   Reduce heat, cover and simmer until liquid is absorbed and rice is still slightly firm. Put the rice mixture into a bowl, add the zucchini and mix. Let cool.

5.   Cut a slice about 1/2 inch (1 cm) on top of the peppers, scoop out and stuff them with the cooled rice mixture. Put the stuffed peppers in slow cooker.

6.   Add water, lemon juice and the remaining oil. Cover and cook on low for 8 hours. To serve, garnish with parsley.

Nutrition Value: Calories: 242, Fat 9g, Carbs 21g, Protein 19.9g

Roasted Potatoes

Servings: 4

Smart Points: 6

Ingredients:
- 4 baking potatoes, well-scrubbed and washed
- 1 c. tablespoons of extra virgin olive oil
- Salt
- 4 sheets of aluminum foil

Directions:
1. Prick the potatoes with a fork in several places.
2. Rub the potatoes with olive oil and sprinkle with salt before wrapping tightly in aluminum foil.
3. Place in a slow cooker, cover and cook on high heat for 4 1/2 to 5 hours, or low heat for 7 1/2- to 8 hours, or until tender.

Nutrition Value: Calories: 230, Fat 9.5g, Carbs 27g, Protein 3.16g

Three Bean Chili

Servings: 6

Smart Points: 5

Ingredients:

- 1 box 28 oz whole tomatoes
- 1/4 cup of tomato paste
- 1 c. to tab chili powder
- 1 c. tsp. dried oregano
- 1 c. tsp. ground cumin
- 1/4 c. tsp. salt
- 1/4 c. tsp. (1 mL) freshly ground black pepper
- 1/4 c. tsp. (1 mL) sugar
- 1 onion, chopped
- 2 cloves finely chopped garlic
- 1 chopped carrot
- 1 chopped celery stalk
- 1 box 19 oz. kidney beans, rinsed and drained
- 1 box 19 oz. black beans, rinsed and drained
- 1 box 19 oz. chickpeas, rinsed and drained

Directions:

1. In slow cooker, using a potato masher, mash the tomatoes.
2. Add tomato paste, chili powder, oregano, cumin, salt, pepper and sugar and mix.
3. Add remaining INGREDIENTS, cover and cook on low for 8 to 10 hours.

Nutrition Value: Calories: 120, Fat 3g, Carbs 31g, Protein 9g

Lentil and Pumpkin Stew

Serve: 6

Smart Points: 4

Ingredients:
- Ground black pepper (to taste)
- Sea salt (to taste)
- Cilantro (1 handful chopped)
- Plain Greek yogurt (.5 cups)
- Nutmeg (1 tsp.)
- Turmeric (1 tsp.)
- Ginger (1 T ground)
- Cumin (1 T ground)
- Lime juice (1 lime)
- Tomato paste (2 T0
- Vegetable broth (4 cups)
- Onion (1 chopped fine)
- Green lentils (1 cup)
- Pumpkin (2 lbs. cubed)

Directions:
- Add the pepper, salt, nutmeg, turmeric, ginger, cumin, lime juice, tomato paste, vegetable broth, onion, green lentils and pumpkin to the slow cooker.
- Cover the slow cooker and let it cook on a low heat for 6 hours.
- Top each serving with plain Greek yogurt and cilantro prior to serving.

Nutrition Value: Calories: 173, Fat 0g, Carbs 32g, Protein 11g

Healthy Vegan Stew

Servings: 10

Smart Points: 3

Ingredients:
- 1 butternut squash
- 1/3 cup raisins
- 1/4 c. chili flakes tea
- 2 cups cubed eggplant
- 1 cup tomato sauce
- 2 cups diced zucchini
- 2 cups frozen okra at room temperature
- 1 cup chopped onion
- 1 ripe tomato, chopped
- 1 thinly sliced carrot
- 1/2 cup vegetable broth
- 1 clove garlic, minced
- 1/2 c. cumin
- 1/2 c. of turmeric
- 1/4 c. cinnamon
- 1/4 c. to paprika

Directions:
1. In a slow cooker, put together the zucchini, okra, squash, eggplant, tomato sauce, carrots, garlic, broth, and raisins.
2. Add the cumin, chili flakes, cinnamon turmeric, and paprika.
3. Cover and cook for 10 hours or until tender vegetables.

Nutrition Value: Calories: 194, Fat 2g, Carbs 16g, Protein 2g

Special Slow Cooker Risotto

Serve: 4

Smart Points: 10

Ingredients:
- Ground black pepper (to taste)
- Sea salt (to taste)
- Lemon zest (1 T0
- Garlic (3 cloves minced)
- Fennel seeds (2 tsp. crushed)
- Plain Greek Yogurt (.3 cups)
- Parmesan cheese (.5 cups grated)
- Mushrooms (.5 cups chopped)
- Shallot (1 finely chopped)
- Carrot (1 peeled, chopped fine)
- Green onions (.3 cups diced)
- Green beans (2 cups cooked)
- Fennel bulb (1 cored, diced fine)
- Dry white wine (.3 cups)
- Water (1 cup)
- Vegetable broth (3 cups)
- Brown rice (1 cup)

Directions:
- Coat the inside of the slow cooker using cooking spray to keep things from sticking.
- Add the garlic, shallot, carrot, rice, fennel and fennel seeds into the slow cooker before adding in the wine, the water and the broth and stirring well.
- Cover the slow cooker and let it cook on a low heat for 3.5 hours.

- Prior to serving, mix in the pepper, lemon zest, yogurt, parmesan cheese, green onions, mushroom and green beans.

Nutrition Value: Calories: 364, Fat 11.8g, Carbs 29g, Protein 29g

Cinnamon Squash and Apples Mix

Servings: 10

Smart Points: 3

Ingredients:

- 1 butternut squash (butternut) 3 lbs, peeled, cored and diced
- 4 apples, peeled, cored and chopped
- 3/4 cup dried cranberries
- 1/2 white onion, chopped (optional)
- 1 c. tablespoon ground cinnamon
- 1 ½ c. with ground nutmeg

Directions:

1. Combine all INGREDIENTS in the bowl of slow cooker.
2. Cook on High heat for 4 hours, or until tender squash. Stir occasionally.

Nutrition Value: Calories: 364, Fat 11.8g, Carbs 29g, Protein 29g

Sweet Potato Soup

Serve: 6
Smart Points: 2

Ingredients:
- Ground black pepper (to taste)
- Sea salt (to taste)
- Dry mustard (1 tsp.)
- Allspice (.5 tsp.)
- Truvia (2 packets)
- Half and half (1.5 cups)
- Sweet potatoes (4 sliced, peeled)
- Vegetable broth (2 cups)

Directions:
- Place the potato slices and the broth into the slow cooker, cover the slow cooker and let it cook on a medium heat for 3 hours.
- Add the results to a food processor and process well.
- Add all of the ingredients to the slow cooker, cover it, and cook at a medium heat for an additional hour.

Nutrition Value: Calories: 112, Fat 1g, Carbs 23g, Protein 2g

Mushroom Vegan Cassoulet

Serving: 9

Smart Points: 8

Ingredients:

- 2 c. tablespoons olive oil
- 1 onion, chopped
- 2 carrots, diced
- 1 lb. of dry white beans
- 4 cups of mushroom broth
- 1 cube of vegetable stock
- 1 bay leaf
- 4 fresh parsley sprigs
- 1 fresh rosemary sprig
- 1 fresh thyme
- 1 branch of fresh savory
- 1 large peeled and cubed potato

Directions:

1. Heat ½ of the olive oil in a skillet and fry the both the onion and carrots until tender.
2. In the bowl of a slow cooker, combine onions, carrots, beans, mushroom broth, bay leaf, and bouillon cube.
3. Add enough water to cover everything completely. Combine the fresh herbs in cheesecloth and add to slow cooker. Cook for 8 hours.
4. Add the potatoes and cook again for 1 hour.
5. Before serving, remove the herbs

Nutrition Value: Calories: 279, Fat 4g, Carbs 47g, Protein 15g

Potato Chowder

Serve: 6

Smart Points: 4

Ingredients:
- Half and half (1 cup)
- Thyme (.25 tsp. crushed)
- Bay leaf (1)
- Barley (.5 cups)
- Vegetable broth (4 cups)
- Garlic (3 cloves minced)
- Leeks (1 cup chopped)
- Carrot (1 diced)
- Potatoes (2 cups cubes)

Directions:
- Place all of the ingredients expect for the half and half into the slow cooker, cover it, and let it cook on a low heat for 6 hours.
- 10 minutes prior to serving, and in the half and half and let it heat, uncovered for 10 minutes.

Nutrition Value: Calories: 170, Fat 2.8g, Carbs 28g, Protein 9g

Soy Sauce Marinated Mushrooms

Servings: 6

Smart Points: 1

Ingredients:
- 2 cups soy sauce
- 2 cups water
- 1 cup butter
- 2 cups sugar
- 4 cups (227 g) white mushrooms

Directions:
1. In a saucepan, combine the soy sauce, water, and butter; Heat over low heat until it melts. Gradually add sugar and stir until dissolved by heating.
2. Place mushrooms in the bowl of the slow cooker and pour the sauce. Cover and cook on low heat (LOW) for 8 to 10 hours, stirring every hour.
3. Refrigerate until ready to serve.

Nutrition Value: Calories: 34.5, Fat 3g, Carbs 3.4g, Protein 1g

Minestrone Soup

Serve: 8
Smart Points: 5

Ingredients:
- Ground black pepper (to taste)
- Sea salt (to taste)
- Parmesan cheese (3 T)
- Extra virgin olive oil (2 T)
- Potato (1 lb., diced, peeled)
- Green beans (1.5 cups chopped)
- Zucchini (1 quartered)
- Leek (1 chopped)
- Celery (1 stalk diced)
- Carrot (1 diced)
- Cannellini beans (19 oz.)
- Tomatoes (14.5 oz. diced)
- Vegetable broth (4 cups)

Directions:
- Add all of the ingredients except for the cheese into the slow cooker and cook, covered, on a low heat for 6 hours.
- Add the parmesan cheese prior to serving.

Nutrition Value: Calories: 250, Fat 3g, Carbs 17g, Protein 2g

Yummy Sweet Vegetable Lasagna

Servings: 6

Smart Points: 8

Ingredients:
- 3 zucchini, sliced 1/2 inch
- 1 eggplant, sliced 1/2 inch
- 1/2 cup tomato sauce or trade
- 1 can (28 oz.) spicy diced tomatoes, drained
- 1/2 can chickpeas
- 1/2 cup spicy salsa
- 275g ricotta
- 1/2 cup grated cheese Italian
- 2 c. olive oil table
- Salt and pepper
- A few arugula leaves
- 1 c. chopped fresh basil

Directions:

1. Coat the bottom of the pot a thin layer of tomato sauce. Spread in a row zucchini. Spray the oil, then sprinkle with salt and pepper.

2. Spread evenly half the ricotta cheese with a spoon. Spread some of the diced tomatoes.

3. Spread in a row the eggplant, then sprinkle with salt and pepper. Repeat with the other half of the ricotta cheese. Spread basil leaves.

4. Spread salsa and chickpeas. Scatter arugula and finish with Italian cheese.

5. Cook 4 1/2 hours at high temperature, or until the cheese is grilled on the sides.

6. When cooking is complete, immediately remove the cover to avoid moisture on top. For the cheese is grilled more, go to the broiler for a few minutes.

Nutrition Value: Calories: 250, Fat 3g, Carbs 17g, Protein 2g

Thyme French Onion Soup

Serve: 6

Smart Points: 10

Ingredients:
- French bread (6 slices)
- Ground black pepper (to taste)
- Sea salt (to taste)
- Goat cheese (2 oz.)
- Vegetable broth (6 cups)
- Thyme (.5 tsp crushed)
- Thyme (3 springs)
- All-purpose flour (1 T)
- Onion (3 lbs. sliced)
- Canola oil (1 T)

Directions:
- Add the oil to a Dutch oven and place it over a medium heat. Add in the salt as well as the onion and let it cook for 35 minutes, stirring regularly.
- Add in the flour and let it cook for 2 minutes, stirring as needed.
- Add the onions into the slow cooker before adding in the pepper as well as the sprigs of thyme. Add in the broth and cook, covered, on a low heat for 10 hours.
- Remove the sprigs of time, plate on top of the bread and then top with the remaining ingredients as desired.

Nutrition Value: Calories: 331, Fat 8g, Carbs 53g, Protein 15g

Delicious Mexican Fried Beans

Servings: 6

Smart Points: 6

Ingredients:
- 1 onion, peeled and halved
- 3 cups red beans, dried, rinsed
- 1/2 jalapeno pepper, seeded and chopped
- 2 c. tablespoons minced garlic
- 5 c. teaspoon salt
- 1 3/4 c. pepper tea
- 1/8 c. ground cumin
- 9 cups water

Directions:
1. Put the onion, beans, jalapeno, garlic, salt, pepper and cumin in a slow cooker.
2. Pour water and stir. Cook on high for 8 hours, adding more water if necessary. NOTE: If more than 1 cup water has evaporated, the temperature is too high.
3. Once the beans are cooked, drain and reserve the liquid. Mash the beans with a potato battery, adding water to achieve desired consistency.

Nutrition Value: Calories: 217, Fat 3g, Carbs 33g, Protein 14g

Conclusion:

Thank you again for purchasing my book! I hope this book was able to provide you with plenty of ideas for recipes that won't just taste good, they will do your body good as well

I hope you've enjoyed this book, and if you don't mind, would you please leave an honest review for this book on Amazon? It'd be greatly appreciated!

Thank you and good luck!

Made in the USA
Lexington, KY
22 November 2017